A Manu...
Emergency Resuscitation

A Manual of Accident and Emergency Resuscitation

Edited by

Colin Robertson and **Keith Little**

*Department of Accident and Emergency Medicine,
Royal Infirmary of Edinburgh*

A Wiley Medical Publication

JOHN WILEY & SONS
Chichester · New York · Brisbane · Toronto · Singapore

Library of Congress Cataloging in Publication Data:
Main entry under title:

A Manual of accident and emergency resuscitation.

   (A Wiley medical publication)
   Bibliography: p.
   Includes index.
   1. Resuscitation — Addresses, essays, lectures.
2. Medical emergencies — Addresses, essays, lectures.
I. Robertson, Colin (Colin Ernest)   II. Little, Keith.
III. Series.
RC86.7.M348   1983   615.8′043   83-1290

ISBN 0 471 90154 7

British Library Cataloguing in Publication Data:

A manual of accident and emergency resuscitation. —
   (Wiley medical publication)
   1. Resuscitation
   I. Robertson, Colin   II. Little, Keith
   615.8′043   RC86.7

ISBN 0 471 90154 7

Phototypeset by Dobbie Typesetting Service, Plymouth, Devon.
Printed by the Pitman Press Limited, Bath, Avon.

CONTENTS

CONTRIBUTORS

DAVID CURRIE, BSc, MBChB, FRCS(Ed), Registrar in Neurosurgery, Royal Infirmary, Aberdeen

CHRISTOPHER HASLETT, BSc(Hons), MBChB, MRCP (UK), Senior Registrar, Department of Medicine, Hammersmith Hospital, London

KEITH LITTLE, MD, Consultant, Department of Accident and Emergency Medicine, Royal Infirmary, Edinburgh

ALASTAIR McGOWAN, BSc, MBChB, MRCP(UK), Registrar in Medicine, Royal Infirmary, Edinburgh

BRIAN POTTER, BSc, MBChB, Registrar, Department of Accident and Emergency Medicine, Royal Infirmary, Edinburgh

SUSAN ROBERTS, MBChB, Registrar, Department of Accident and Emergency Medicine, Royal Infirmary, Edinburgh

COLIN ROBERTSON, MBChB, MRCP(UK), Senior Registrar, Department of Accident and Emergency Medicine, Royal Infirmary, Edinburgh

SUSAN STEELE, BSc, MBChB, Registrar, Department of Accident and Emergency Medicine, Royal Infirmary, Edinburgh

ACKNOWLEDGEMENT

We wish to acknowledge Christine Mitchell and Lindsay Robertson for their help in preparation of the manuscript and Daphne Lytton for providing the illustrations.

Fig. 7 is adapted, with permission, from the Therapeutic Schedule, Coronary Care Unit, Royal Infirmary, Edinburgh.

INTRODUCTION

The Junior Casualty Officer may be faced with life-threatening situations where prompt and appropriate management is required before the assistance of senior experienced colleagues can be obtained. This manual aims to cover the recognition, investigations, and *immediate* care needed for the common life-threatening emergencies in adult patients presenting to the Accident and Emergency Department.

It must be emphasized that there is no substitute for experience in such cases. The guidelines expressed are necessarily brief and dogmatic. No apology is offered for this, since in the heat of the moment clear concise instructions are more valuable than a longer technical discussion of the problems. However, the reader is strongly advised to consult the books and articles mentioned on page 174 for detailed discussion of the various conditions presented here. In addition, the Casualty Officer should obtain experience in the performance of the techniques described in section 4 at leisure under expert guidance.

Finally, when in doubt, *call for help*. The correct care of a patient in such circumstances is more important

than an attempt to muddle through in order to preserve
false pride.

COLIN ROBERTSON
KEITH LITTLE
Edinburgh, 1983

Section I

CARDIOPULMONARY RESUSCITATION

DIAGNOSIS OF CARDIAC ARREST

- Loss of consciousness, together with:
- Absent femoral or carotid pulses.

Note

- Observations of pupillary changes, respiration or colour change are unreliable and waste time.
- The diagnosis of 'cardiac arrest' is a *clinical* one; treat the patient, *not* the electrocardiogram monitor trace.

MANAGEMENT

- Place the patient on a hard surface. If patient is on the floor do not waste time lifting him onto a trolley.
- Strike the patient once over mid/lower sternum with a firm blow.
- Commence cardiac massage. Using two-handed technique, apply compression over the lower sternum at a rate of 50–60 compressions per minute.
- Ensure airway (see page 26) and commence ventilation by either:
  - Mouth-to-mouth.
  - Brooks airway.

- •Guedal airway.
- •Endotracheal intubation and intermittent positive pressure ventilation (IPPV).
- •Insert an i.v. cannula (preferably via a central route if experienced in this technique). Run in 100 ml 8.4% sodium bicarbonate immediately to correct the associated acidosis and give further aliquots as necessary following arterial blood gas sampling.
- •Apply a 200 J direct current shock as soon as possible.
- •Establish electrocardiographic monitoring, observe electrocardiograph trace and administer rational treatment for arrhythmia(s) (see page 6).

Throughout resuscitation

- •Interruptions in cardiac massage and ventilation (e.g. for the purposes of intubation/defibrillation, etc.) must never exceed 15 seconds.
- •Periodically check for carotid or femoral pulses both during and without cardiac massage.
- •Check pupillary responses to light.
- •Check whether oxygenation and correction of acidosis is adequate (repeat arterial blood gases every 10 minutes if possible).
- •Perform frequent bronchial toilet.
- •Cardiac massage and ventilation must be continuously performed until an adequate spontaneous cardiac

output and ventilation are achieved or the decision to discontinue resuscitation is made.

When cardiac output is regained

- Treat the underlying arrhythmia rationally (see page 6).
- Obtain a chest x-ray and look for rib or sternal fractures or pneumothorax secondary to the resuscitation.

If attempts at resuscitation are unsuccessful consider the following possibilities

- Electrolyte disturbance.
- Inadequate or overcorrection of acidosis.
- Adequate circulating blood volume.
- Pneumothorax or cardiac tamponade.
- Overdosage or associated toxic drug effects, e.g. digoxin, or tricyclic antidepressant drugs.

The decision to abandon resuscitation is unique for each patient and should preferably be made by a senior doctor. Factors influencing the decision may, however, include:

- The patient's age and underlying diseases or conditions. (In younger patients and in hypothermic or poisoned

patients, resuscitative efforts should be continued for relatively longer periods.)
- The duration of the cardiac arrest and response to cardiopulmonary resuscitation.
- Electromechanical dissociation.

ARRHYTHMIAS

GENERAL PRINCIPLES

- Treat the patient, *not* the cardiac monitor trace. Ensure that an 'arrhythmia' is not due to faults in the electrodes or monitoring equipment.
- Throughout the procedure(s), ensure that the patient's airway is clear, and that he is adequately oxygenated, has a cardiac monitor attached, and defibrillation/resuscitation equipment is immediately to hand.
- All patients should have an i.v. cannula *in situ* to provide immediate i.v. access.
- Remember that in patients with arrhythmias causing a reduced cardiac output, circulation times for drugs given intravenously will be prolonged.
- Avoid polypharmacy.
- Consider the possibility of acid–base or electrolyte disturbances as a cause for arrhythmias, or for their failure to respond to treatment.

•Following the emergency treatment of all arrhythmias, the patient should be referred for specialist care.

SPECIFIC ARRHYTHMIAS

ASYSTOLE

Clinical features

•'Cardiac arrest'.

Electrocardiographic features

•'Straight line' electrocardiogram.

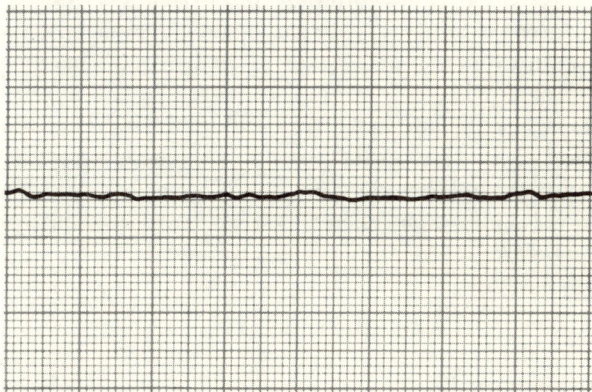

Fig. 1.

8

Management

- Commence cardiopulmonary resuscitation (see page 3).
- Administer: isoprenaline 100 μg followed by 10% calcium gluconate 20 ml, i.v. (preferably via a central vein).
- If there is no response to these drugs continue cardiopulmonary resuscitation and progressively take the following steps as required:
  - Give 1 ml of adrenaline 1:1000 i.v.
  - If a central i.v. line is *in situ*, give a further bolus of 1 ml adrenaline 1:100 followed by 10 ml of 10% calcium gluconate. If only a peripheral i.v. line is present, give these drugs by the intracardiac route.
  - Insert a temporary (transvenous, oesophageal, or transthoracic) pacemaker if experienced in these techniques.
- Occasionally the above steps will result in the restoration of a stable cardiac rhythm with adequate cardiac output; however, more commonly, ventricular fibrillation is induced and should then be treated appropriately as below.

VENTRICULAR FIBRILLATION

Clinical features

- 'Cardiac arrest'.

Electrocardiographic features

• Chaotic electrical activity.

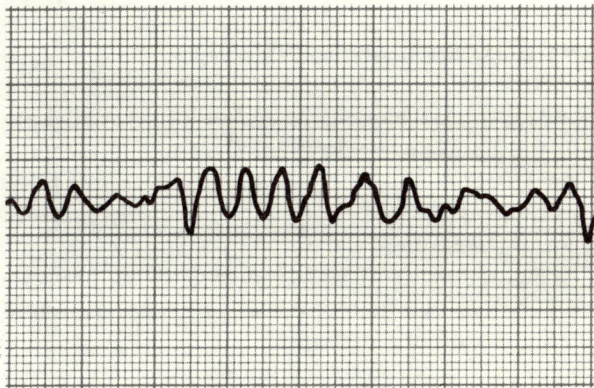

Fig. 2

Management

• Commence cardiopulmonary resuscitation (see page 3).
• Administer an immediate d.c. shock with an energy of 200 J.
• If there is no response, or if ventricular fibrillation recurs after a short period:
  • Give 100 mg lignocaine i.v. as a bolus, then repeat the d.c. shock at 400 J.

- Repeat the above step.
- Give 150 mg mexiletine i.v. as a bolus and repeat the d.c. shock.
- If ventricular fibrillation is persistently of low amplitude, then give 100 μg isoprenaline i.v. to 'coarsen' the ventricular fibrillation and then repeat the d.c. shock at 400 J.
- Recheck arterial blood gases and seek further advice:
  - Is the associated acidosis corrected and oxygenation adequate?
  - Is there any reason to suspect an electrolyte disturbance? (Check urea and electrolytes.)
  - Is digoxin toxicity likely? If so, give 100 mg phenytoin i.v. (which can be repeated if necessary) as a bolus prior to further d.c. shocks.
- When a rhythm resulting in an adequate cardiac output is restored, start an infusion of lignocaine (1.5 g lignocaine in 500 ml 5% dextrose administered at 80 ml/h for the first 30 minutes then 40 ml/h for the next 2 hours.

VENTRICULAR TACHYCARDIA

Clinical features

- Usually presents with signs of 'cardiac arrest' or low cardiac output (see page 39).

•Cannon waves may be visible in the jugular venous pulse and the first heart sounds may have a varying intensity.

Electrocardiographic features

•Broad aberrant QRS complexes which are usually not entirely regular and not all of identical shape.
•Random P waves may be seen.

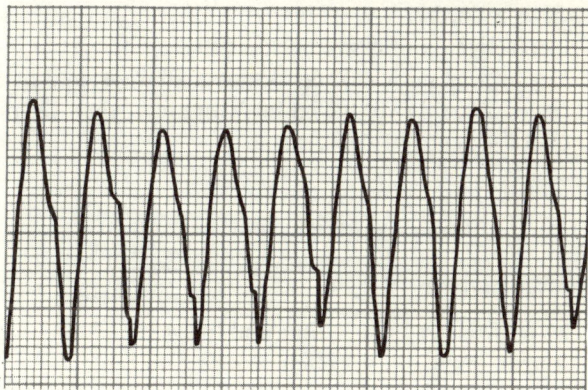

Fig. 3

Management

- Usually d.c. shock (100–200 J) is required.
  - Immediately if the patient is unconscious, or:
  - After administration of a general anaesthetic or i.v. sedation from an anaesthetic specialist.
- If the arrhythmia is refractory:
  - Give 100 mg lignocaine i.v. and repeat the d.c. shock. Commence a lignocaine infusion (1.5 g lignocaine in 500 ml 5% dextrose administered at a rate of 80 ml/h for first 30 minutes then 40 ml/h for the next 2 hours).
- If ventricular tachycardia recurs:
  - Give a further i.v. bolus of 100 mg lignocaine. If ineffective: commence an i.v. infusion of mexiletine (1 g mexiletine in 500 ml dextrose administered at a rate of 125 ml over the initial 30 minutes, then 125 ml over the next 150 minutes).

ATRIAL FIBRILLATION

Clinical features

- The pulse is irregular in time and force.
- An apex–radial pulse deficit may be detectable.
- With very rapid or slow ventricular rates, features of a low cardiac output may be present.

Electrocardiographic features

• The baseline trace is chaotic with no visible P waves and an irregular ventricular rate.

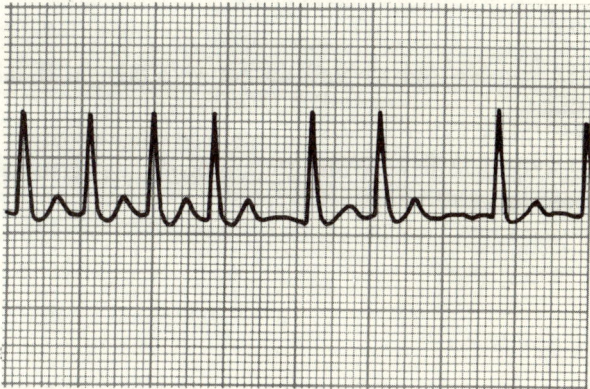

Fig. 4

Management

• Treatment is not immediately required unless the patient has features of low cardiac output, in which case d.c. shock (energy required usually 20–50 J) under general anaesthetic or i.v. sedation administered by an anaesthetic specialist should be given.

- If the patient is well and has not had digitalis-like drugs recently, give digoxin (0.5 mg digoxin in 50 ml 5% dextrose administered over 10–15 minutes as an i.v. infusion).

Note

Seek specialist advice and do not give digoxin if the patient:
- May have digitalis toxicity or is already digitalized.
- Is known to have Wolff–Parkinson–White (or other accessory pathway) syndrome.

ATRIAL FLUTTER

Clinical features

- The pulse rate may be irregular or regular (commonly at a rate of 150/min).
- 'Flutter waves' may be seen in the jugular venous pulse.

Electrocardiographic features

- The ventricular rate is commonly regular at 150/min (2:1 atrioventricular block). However, other degrees of atrioventricular block (1:1, 3:1, 4:1, etc.) can occur.

- Atrial 'flutter waves' may be visible or demonstrated more clearly if slowing of the ventricular rate by carotid sinus massage is produced.

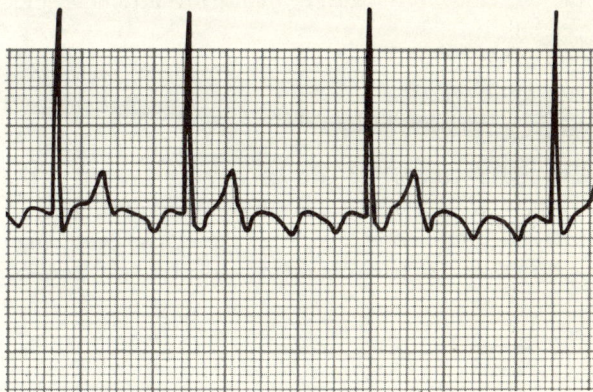

Fig. 5

Management

- As for atrial fibrillation.

SUPRAVENTRICULAR AND PAROXYSMAL ATRIAL TACHYCARDIAS

Clinical features

- The heart rate may be 140/min or more, but is often well tolerated by the patient.
- Carotid sinus massage may terminate the arrhythmia, or increase any degree of atrioventricular block present.

Electrocardiographic features

- The QRS complexes are usually narrow (less than 3 mm). If aberrant atrioventricular conduction is present, broad complexes similar to those occurring in ventricular tachycardia may be present; however,

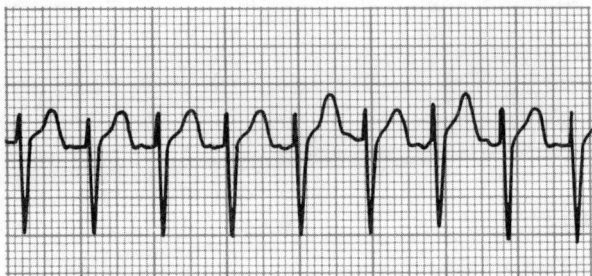

Fig. 6

every QRS complex is identical and the rhythm is usually regular.
●If P waves are visible they are associated with the QRS complexes.

Management

Supraventricular tachycardia / paroxysmal atrial tachycardia

Apply carotid sinus massage

Arrhythmia persists | Arrhythmia terminated

Well tolerated by patients | Mild hypotension present | Circulatory failure

Refer for definitive treatment | Is patient on digoxin or β-blocking agent | Immediate d.c. cardioversion | Refer for maintenance therapy

Yes | No

Give i.v. practolol | Give i.v. verapamil

Terminates arrhythmia | No effect

Refer for maintenance therapy | Refer for elective d.c. cardioversion

No effect

Seek further advice

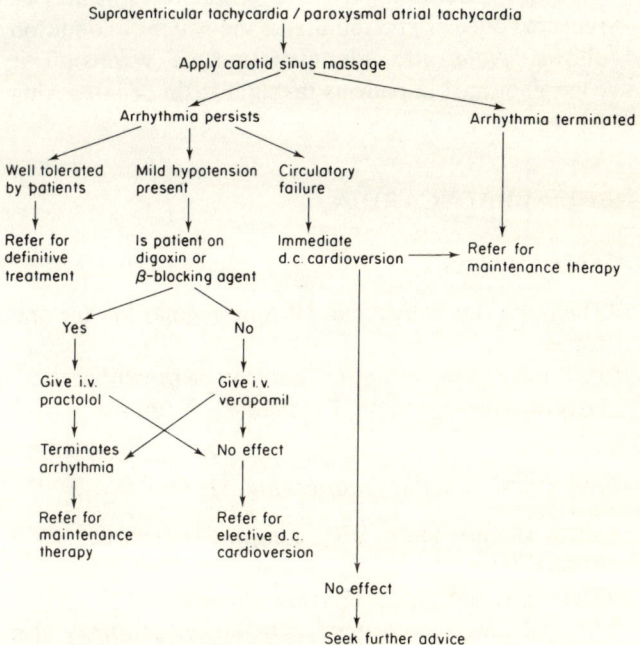

Fig. 7. Management of supraventricular tachycardia/paroxysmal atrial tachycardia

Drug doses

- *Practolol:* given 5 mg i.v. over 5 minutes. Wait and observe for 5 minutes with regular checks of patient's condition. The dose can be repeated up to a total dose of 15 mg.
- *Verapamil:* Give 5 mg i.v. over 5 minutes; this may be repeated once after 5 minutes if the patient's condition allows. *Note:* the administration of verapamil is contraindicated in patients taking digoxin or β-blocking agents.

SINUS BRADYCARDIA

Clinical features

- The pulse rate is less than 60/min, regular in time and force.
- Features of low cardiac output may be present particularly at ventricular rates less than 40–50/min.

Electrocardiographic features (Fig. 8)

- Sinus rhythm (each QRS complex is preceded by a normal P wave).
- The ventricular rate is less than 60/min.
- An associated respiratory sinus arrhythmia may also be present.

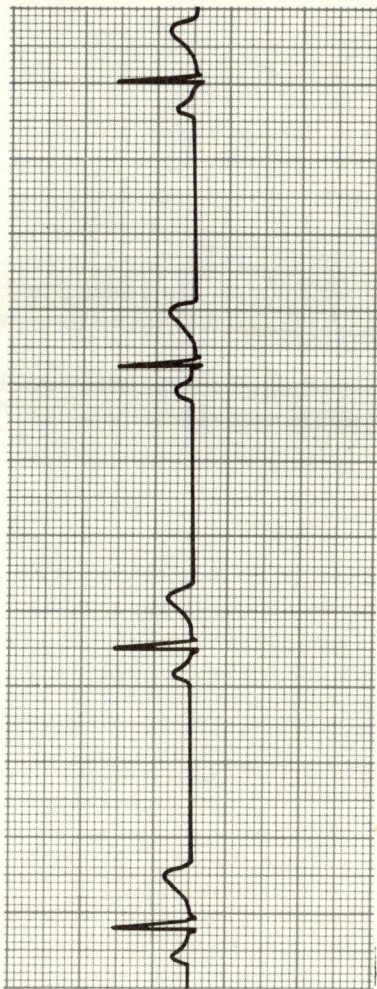

Fig. 8

Management

● Usually no specific therapy is necessary unless:
  ● The arrhythmia is not tolerated by the patient.
  ● Ventricular 'escape' arrhythmias occur.
● If required, give:
  ● Atropine as an i.v. bolus (dose 0.6–1.8 mg).
  ● If there is no response, an isoprenaline infusion or the insertion of a temporary pacemaker may rarely be required.

Note: if the sinus bradycardia is related to β-blocker toxicity see page 143.

HEART BLOCK

The clinical features of heart block depend principally upon their effect on the ventricular rate; however, at ventricular rates less than 50/min, symptoms related to consequent low cardiac output are often present.

Electrocardiographic features

First degree heart block (Fig. 9)
● The P–R interval is greater than 0.20 seconds.
● The QRS complex morphology is normal.

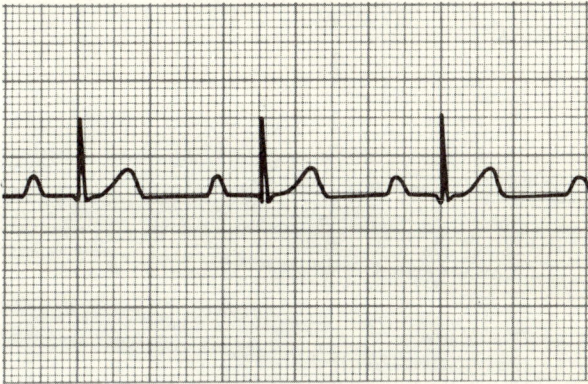

Fig. 9

Second degree heart block
•P waves occur regularly but are not all followed by QRS complexes. This may take the form of a progressive lengthening of the P–R interval until a QRS complex is dropped (Fig. 10a). Alternatively the P–R interval may remain constant, but intermittently QRS complexes are absent (Figs. 10b, 11).

Third degree heart block (Fig. 12)
•P waves and QRS complexes are present, but occur independently.

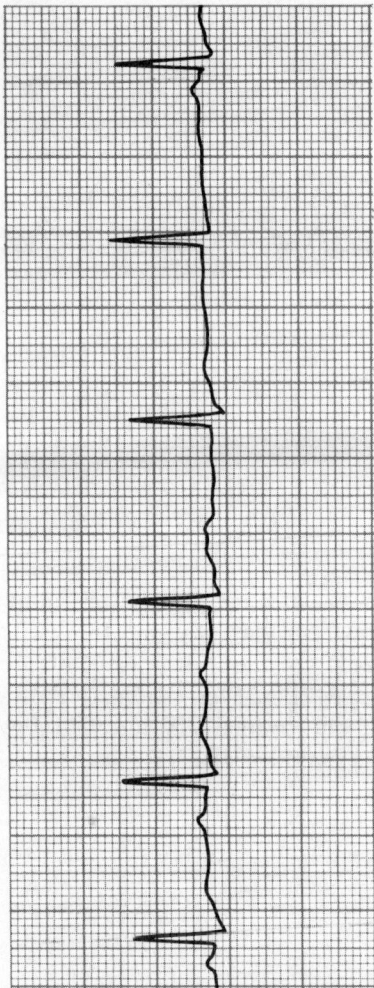

Fig. 10a

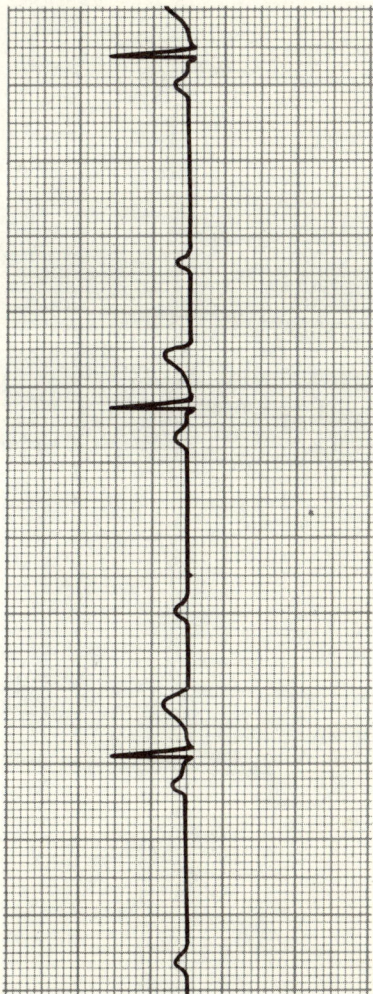

Fig. 10b

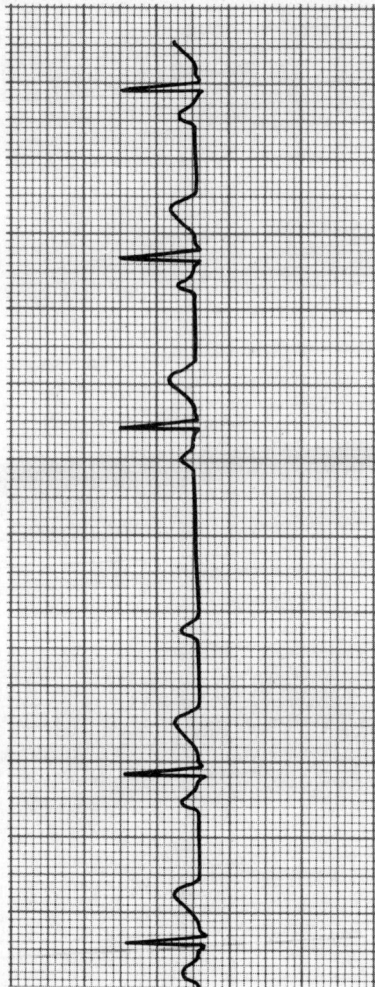

Fig. 11

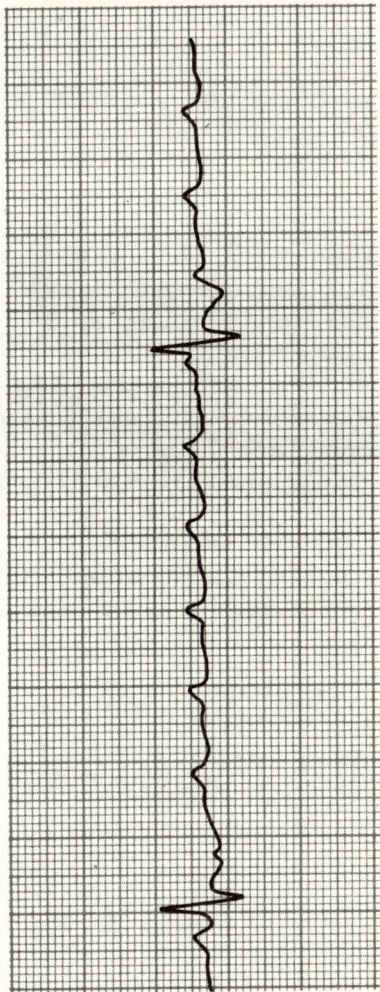

Fig. 12

●The QRS morphology may be normal, or widened depending upon the site of ventricular activation.

Management

●If symptoms are present, and are related to brady-cardia as a consequence of heart block, increases in the ventricular rate may be induced by the following measures:
  ·Administration of i.v. atropine (dose: 0.6–1.8 mg).
  ·Administration of an isoprenaline infusion (dose: 2 mg of isoprenaline in 500 ml of 5% dextrose contains 4 μg/ml. The infusion rate should commence at 0.5–1 μg/min initially. In the absence of any clinical response or ventricular tachyarrhythmias the infusion rate may be increased to 10–15 μg/min if required).
  ·The insertion of a temporary cardiac pacemaker.

AIRWAY CARE

COMMON CAUSES OF AIRWAY OBSTRUCTION

●Loss of muscle tone, particularly when the patient is lying flat, will result in the tongue falling back against the palate.
●Foreign matter in the upper or lower airway, e.g.

blood, vomit, secretions, teeth, and other foreign bodies.
- Laryngospasm, laryngeal oedema, epiglottitis, pseudo-membrane, etc.
- Dysfunction of a mechanical ventilatory aid, e.g. blocked endotracheal tube.
- Note that severe bronchospasm or a tension pneumo-thorax can mimic the clinical features of severe acute airway obstruction.

RECOGNITION OF AIRWAY OBSTRUCTION

- Absent or noisy airflow: the character of airway noises may suggest the site(s) of obstruction, viz.:
  - 'Snoring' — tongue against palate.
  - 'Gargling' — secretions, vomit, blood in oropharynx.
  - Stridor — laryngeal/upper airway obstruction.
  - 'Wheezing' — lower airway/bronchial obstruction.
- If spontaneous respiration is present, associated features may include:
  - Vigorous abdominal wall movement.
  - Intercostal muscle indrawing and use of other accessory muscles of respiration.
  - Tracheal 'tug'.
- Cyanosis and/or impairment of conscious level may occur, but are *not* good indicators of adequacy of ventilation.

- Resistance to inflation during positive pressure ventilation.

MANAGEMENT OF AIRWAY OBSTRUCTION

General points

- Clear any debris from the mouth and oropharynx manually and using a suction catheter.
- The head should be extended on the neck with the lower jaw pulled anteriorly.
- If the patient is breathing spontaneously with an apparently clear airway:
  - Place the patient in the semi-prone position.
  - Administer a high concentration (40–60%) of inspired oxygen via face mask.
  - Constantly reassess the need for further measures (see below).
- If the airway appears to remain obstructed, consider the possibility of tracheal occlusion due to an impacted foreign body; this commonly presents as a 'choking' patient, who is cyanosed, cannot speak and is clutching his neck.
- If possible, the patient should attempt to clear his airway spontaneously by coughing. If this is not possible or unsuccessful, perform the Heimlich manoeuvre.

- If there is no response and attempts to remove the foreign body under direct vision are unsuccessful seek urgent specialist advice, and if necessary, perform cricothyrotomy (see below) while preparations are made for skilled tracheostomy.
- The use of an oropharyngeal airway in a patient with altered consciousness will provide access for suction, but does not alone provide definitive airway care. In addition, inappropriate usage may provoke vomiting and/or laryngospasm.

ENDOTRACHEAL INTUBATION

The technique can only be learned by practice under skilled supervision, although mannikin and/or cadaver practice is useful.

Indications

- Endotracheal intubation may be required in a patient with:
  - Absence of spontaneous respiration.
  - Altered consciousness and loss of protective airway reflexes.
  - A special need for ventilation, tracheal access or protection, e.g. head injury, severe pulmonary oedema.

Procedure

- Always have suction apparatus and an introducer *immediately* to hand.
- Use a lubricated endotracheal tube, the cuff of which has been checked for leakage. The tube should be cut to the appropriate length prior to use. Commonly used endotracheal tube sizes are:
  - Adult male: 8.5–9.5 mm
  - Adult female: 7.5–8.5 mm
- Position the patient's head on a pillow, causing the neck to be slightly flexed and extend the head on the neck.
- Using a curved-blade laryngoscope held in the left hand, introduce the blade to the right of the tongue and note the following landmarks:
  - Tonsillar column.
  - Epiglottis.
  - Vallecula.
- Place the tip of the blade in the vallecula and using a straight lift, expose the vocal cords by pulling the laryngoscope anteriorly.
- Under direct vision, pass the endotracheal tube through the vocal cords into the trachea.
- Inflate the cuff until no air leakage occurs during ventilation and tie/tape the tube securely in place.

Following insertion

- Check the position of the tube by auscultating both sides of the chest during ventilation and ensure that air entry is equal.
- Obtain a chest x-ray to confirm adequate positioning.

Complications of endotracheal intubation

- Trauma to lips, tongue, teeth, and vocal cords may be caused by poor technique (particularly by pivoting the laryngoscope against the patient's upper teeth).
- Inadvertent intubation of the oesophagus or right main bronchus are uncommon provided scrupulous attention is paid to technique.
- Coughing, bronchospasm, laryngospasm, and arrhythmias may be provoked by oropharyngeal stimulation.

EXTUBATION

- The patient should be well oxygenated and the bronchial tree and pharynx aspirated prior to removal. The endotracheal tube should be withdrawn gently and smoothly.
- Further suction and the administration of a high concentration (40–60%) of oxygen via face mask should be provided as necessary.

CRICOTHYROTOMY

•If immediate access to a patient's airway is required and endotracheal intubation is impossible or inadvisable, cricothyrotomy may 'buy time' while urgent preparations for skilled tracheostomy are being made.

Technique

•The patient should be supine with the head extended on the neck.
•Hold the larynx between the thumb and middle finger and identify the cricothyroid membrane by palpation.
•Insert two large-bore cannulae (12–14G) percutaneously

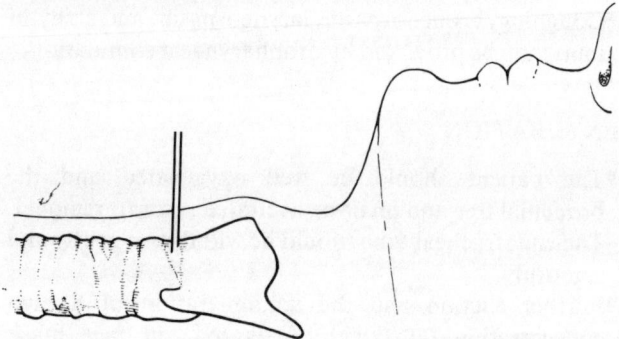

Fig. 13. Cannula position for cricothyrotomy

through the cricothyroid membrane into the trachea (Fig. 13).
- Place a suitable oxygen mask (which will deliver a high concentration of inspired oxygen) over the cannulae.

Possible problems

- Insufflation of soft tissues with air or tracheal damage may occur but are uncommon provided the cannulae are inserted with care.

THE SHOCKED PATIENT

RECOGNITION

The shocked patient will have some or all of the following features:
- Hypotension—systolic blood pressure less than 90 mmHg (*or*, a fall in systolic blood pressure of 40 mmHg or more in an elderly or previously hypertensive patient).
- Reduced skin perfusion—the skin is cool, clammy, and pale with delay in capillary filling (greater than 2 seconds). In early 'septic' shock, however, the patient's skin may be warm and pink due to peripheral vasodilatation.

- Reduced cerebral perfusion—may present as confusion, restlessness, or altered consciousness.
- Reduced renal perfusion—oliguria (less than 50 ml urine/hour).

CLINICAL TYPES

HYPOVOLAEMIC SHOCK

This is the commonest type encountered in the Accident and Emergency Department and may be due to:
- Reduced circulating blood volume:
  - Traumatic blood loss:
    - Overt, e.g. open wound(s), arterial bleeding.
    - Occult, e.g. blunt abdominal trauma, haemothorax, closed limb fractures.
  - Gastrointestinal blood loss, e.g. haematemesis, melaena.
- Reduced plasma volume:
  - Plasma loss, e.g. burns, pancreatitis.
  - Water and electrolyte loss, e.g. diarrhoea, vomiting, burns, heat stroke, Addison's disease, diabetes.

Management

Airway
- Ensure an adequate airway (see page 26).

• Administer as high an inspired concentration of oxygen as possible.

Obvious blood loss
• Apply direct pressure.
• Clamp arterial bleeding points.

i.v. access
• In general, at least one large bore (14 or 16G) peripheral line and one central venous line will be initially required.
• The number of further i.v. lines set up will vary depending upon severity of the clinical situation.
• At the time the i.v. line is inserted, blood should be withdrawn and sent for grouping and cross-matching.
• If any plasma expander or blood has been previously given, e.g. in transit to hospital, inform the Blood Transfusion Service.

Assessment of blood/extracellular fluid deficits

Traumatic blood loss
Very rough approximations for a 70 kg man (in whom total circulatory blood volume is approximately 5 litres) are:

Arm/lower leg fractures	500–1500 ml/fracture
Femur	1000–2000 ml/fracture

Closed injuries of pelvis,
abdomen, or chest   1000–4000 ml each

Burns (see page 76)

Volume (in ml) required over initial 4–6 hour period since injury	=	Percentage area of burn	×	Body weight (in kg)

Water and electrolyte loss
The presence of clinical signs of water and electrolyte depletion (skin turgor, dry tongue, reduced eyeball tension, etc.) implies at least a loss of 5% of total body extracellular fluid, i.e. 2–3 litres in a 70 kg man.

Investigations
- Send venous blood sample for estimation of urea and electrolytes.
- Check arterial blood gases.
- Chest x-ray.
- Test urine for blood, glucose, and ketones.

Monitor and record the following parameters
(initially every 5 minutes)
- Heart rate (from cardiac monitor).
- Blood pressure (remember that at low blood pressures, electronic sphygmomanometers are often inaccurate).
- Central venous pressure.

Further procedures

- Pass a urinary catheter. Measure residual bladder volume and hourly urine output.
- Pass a nasogastric tube and aspirate stomach contents.
- Consider applying Newcastle G-suit or military anti-shock trousers in the following situations:
  - Major abdominal trauma.
  - Pelvic fractures.
  - Lower limb fractures.

These devices:
  - Autotransfuse 500–1000 ml blood into systemic circulation.
  - Tamponade bleeding vessels/surfaces.
  - Prevent examination of abdomen, pelvis, and legs.
  - May act to splint diaphragm and embarrass ventilation.
  - Must not be deflated except in theatre with a surgical team ready to operate and with rapid i.v. replacement possible.

The choice of i.v. fluid therapy in hypovolaemic shock

This is a highly controversial area. We suggest the following sequential regimen:
- 1000 ml 0.9% saline/Ringer lactate solution, followed by:
- 1000 ml dextran 70 in 0.9% saline.

- While awaiting blood, continue with 0.9% saline.
  Blood transfusion:
  - Usually type specific or O—ve blood will be supplied by the Blood Transfusion Service.
  - Use blood warmers and filters if possible.
  - Give 10 ml of 10% calcium gluconate for each litre of blood given.
  - If more than 8 units of blood are required or given, a coagulation screen should be performed and specialist haematological advice sought, as platelet transfusions and/or fresh frozen plasma may be required.

Note

- The volume of the infusion given is more important than its content.
- Individual readings of pulse rate, blood pressure, and central venous pressure can be misleading; the *frequent* measurement of these parameters and their trends are far more reliable as an indication of therapeutic response.
- If more than 2–3 litres of i.v. fluid have been given with no change in vital signs, then either the patient requires blood transfusion or the diagnosis of hypovolaemic shock *alone* is wrong.
- If, after estimated volume losses have been replaced, the blood pressure remains low and the central

venous pressure is high (greater than $10\,cmH_2O$) consider:

- •Is the central venous line correctly positioned (check a penetrated chest x-ray) and swinging freely with respiration?
- •Is there a primary or secondary myocardial problem resulting in a low-output state, e.g. cardiac tamponade, myocardial infarction, ischaemia or contusion?
- •If the central venous line is correctly positioned and the possibility of cardiac tamponade is excluded, then specialist advice regarding the use of an inotropic agent (e.g. dopamine, dobutamine) should be obtained.

●The administration of high-dose corticosteroids or digoxin has no proven value in the initial resuscitation of patients with hypovolaemic shock.

CARDIOGENIC SHOCK

This state implies a low or inadequate cardiac output due to a primary cardiac problem. In addition to the recognized features of shock (as above), patients with cardiogenic shock may have:
●Elevated jugular venous pressure.
●Signs of pulmonary oedema.
●Soft heart sounds, extra heart sounds, precordial thrills or murmurs.

Causes

- Acute myocardial infarction is by far the commonest cause. A history of chest pain or collapse may be obtained. The electrocardiogram will commonly show acute changes of infarction or severe ischaemia.
- Papillary muscle or septal rupture may occur several days following acute myocardial infarction. A loud systolic murmur/thrill may be heard at the lower left sternal edge.
- Myocardial contusion—related to chest trauma.
- Obstructed or malfunctioning artificial heart valves.
- Pericardial tamponade—related to trauma, myocardial infarction with ventricular rupture, or (rarely) pericarditis.
- Major pulmonary embolism.

Investigations

- 12 lead electrocardiogram
- Chest x-ray.
- Urea and electrolytes.
- Arterial blood gases.

Management

Airway
Give a high concentration (40–60%) of inspired oxygen via face mask.

i.v. access
A peripheral i.v. cannula should be inserted and either
flushed with heparinized saline and occluded, or kept
open with a slow-running infusion of 5% dextrose.

Cardiac monitor

Analgesia
If required, give morphine i.v. in 2.5 mg aliquots,
cautiously titrated to response.

Arrhythmias
Brady- or tachyarrhythmias, causing a low cardiac
output state, will require urgent therapy (see page 6).

Metabolic disturbance
Hypoxia, acid–base, and electrolyte disturbances
should be appropriately corrected under specialist
advice.

SEPTIC SHOCK

This is an uncommon, frequently unrecognized
condition. In addition to the recognized clinical features
of shock, the septic patient may also have:
●Pyrexia, a history of chills, rigors, or symptoms
  related to focus of infection.
●Warm, pink extremities (although capillary filling is
  still delayed) due to peripheral vasodilatation.

- Skin rashes (especially in meningo-, strepto- or staphy-lococcal septicaemias).
- Evidence of disseminated intravascular coagulation: bruising, petechial haemorrhages, spontaneous bleeding from mucous membranes/gastrointestinal tract, oozing from venepuncture sites.
- Mild icterus.
- Electrocardiogram abnormalities (non-specific ST–T wave changes and supraventricular arrhythmias, in particular atrial fibrillation, are common).

Investigations

Take and send the appropriate blood samples for:
- Arterial blood gas analysis.
- Plasma urea, electrolyte, calcium, and glucose measurements.
- Full blood count and coagulation screen.
  - Grouping and cross-matching.
  - Blood cultures.
- Chest x-ray.
- Electrocardiogram.

Management

Airway and ventilation
Septicaemic patients are commonly hypoxic. This may be adequately corrected by increasing the inspired

oxygen concentration, via face mask, but may require intubation and assisted ventilation.

Correction of fluid, electrolyte, and acid–base abnormalities
● 'Blind' intravenous therapy may be hazardous. These patients may have pulmonary oedema related to acute cardiac, renal, or respiratory failure. For this reason, the measurement of central venous pressure is valuable.

If the central venous pressure is low (less than + 5 cmH$_2$O), 500 ml 0.9% saline should be infused over 30 minutes and the response of vital signs and the central venous pressure closely monitored.

If the central venous pressure is high (greater than + 15 cmH$_2$O), pulmonary oedema, pneumothorax, or bronchospasm should be excluded.
● Metabolic disturbances—chiefly hypo- or hyper-kalaemia, hypocalcaemia, and hypoglycaemia are common and should be treated appropriately.
● Associated acid–base disturbances may also require correction and specialist advice should be sought.

Drug therapy
● This has little role in the initial resuscitation of the septicaemic patient.
● 'Blind' antibiotic therapy may confuse further bacteriological investigations and aggravate the clinical

picture (e.g. by liberating large amounts of circulating endotoxin).

- If despite the correction of ventilatory, fluid, electrolyte, and acid–base disturbances, the patient remains hypotensive and the clinical situation is deteriorating, then seek specialist advice regarding the possible use of high-dose corticosteroids, inotropic agents, etc.

Section 2

HEAD INJURY

GENERAL POINTS

- The early management of injuries causing respiratory embarrassment or shock is essential to the successful treatment of the head injury.
- Patients with head injury and disturbed consciousness commonly have other associated injuries, in particular of cervical spine, chest, and pelvis. These injuries may not be apparent on clinical examination alone.
- Absence of clinical or radiological evidence of head injury does not exclude traumatic intracranial pathology as a cause of altered consciousness.
- Specialist advice must be sought early if a patient exhibits:
  - Neurological deterioration (see page 53)
  - Localizing neurological signs.
- Consider whether the head injury may be secondary to a prior event, e.g. cerebrovascular accident, epileptic fit, hypoglycaemia.
- Remember the possibility of head injury in all cases of altered consciousness or behavioural disturbance.

THE FULLY CONSCIOUS PATIENT

History and examination should be directed towards identifying those patients at risk of developing

48

complications (e.g. intracranial haematoma, infection, post-concussional syndrome).

History

- Period of loss of consciousness or post-traumatic amnesia.
- Headache, increasing drowsiness, visual disturbance, fitting, or vomiting.

Examination

- A full neurological examination is mandatory.
- Baseline observations should be recorded (preferably on the Glasgow coma chart).
- Look for periorbital or subconjunctival haematomata.
- Look for blood and/or cerebrospinal fluid leakage from ears and nose. (In the absence of bleeding, cerebrospinal fluid may be distinguished from nasal secretions by testing for glucose content with reagent strips.)
- Examine the scalp thoroughly for lacerations, bruising, and 'boggy' areas.

X-rays

Good quality radiographs are essential and should include the following views:

- Anteroposterior.
- Lateral.
- Towne's.

Note: every patient with altered consciousness must be accompanied by a doctor or nurse during x-ray procedures.

Management

Local injury

- Scalp lacerations can bleed profusely. If there is significant blood loss, admission for transfusion may be required.
- After thorough cleansing/débridement, simple linear scalp lacerations should be sutured in one layer to achieve local haemostasis.
- Whenever suturing scalp lacerations, the underlying bony surface should be palpated to exclude associated fracture.

Skull fractures

- The majority of intracranial haematomata are associated with radiological evidence of skull fracture.
- However, base of skull fractures may *not* be radiologically apparent on the standard views. Their presence is suggested by periorbital/subconjunctival haemorrhage, bleeding or cerebrospinal fluid leakage from ears or nose.

- In patients with compound skull fractures, the overlying wound should merely be dressed until the area can be fully explored in theatre.
- An intracranial aerocele complicating a compound fracture can only be excluded by a supine lateral skull x-ray.

Referral

Patients should be referred for observation/admission if there is:
- A history of loss of consciousness.
- Post-traumatic amnesia, a state of altered consciousness or neurological abnormality or symptoms.
- Skull fracture(s).

During referral and transfer of the patient, neurological observations should be continued.

THE PATIENT WITH ALTERED CONSCIOUSNESS

- The prevention/treatment of concomitant respiratory embarrassment and hypovolaemia will reduce the possibility of secondary cerebral damage.
- The recognition and treatment of other injuries (in particular to cervical spine, chest, and pelvis) should be remembered.

History

- Ask ambulancemen, police and attendants specifically about:
  - Mechanism of injury.
  - Initial state of consciousness and subsequent changes.
  - Evidence of vomiting or aspiration.

Examination

- Whenever a traumatized patient with an altered state of consciousness is moved or examined, the possibility of an associated spinal fracture should be considered.
- Head and neck movement should be prevented either by manual control or the application of a cervical collar.
- A full neurological examination is mandatory.
- Neurological observations should initially be performed and recorded every 5 minutes (on the Glasgow coma chart).
- A brief, but thorough, examination of the chest, abdomen, pelvis, and limbs should follow.

Management

Airway

- The establishment of an adequate airway, with correction of hypoxia, hypercapnia, and acidosis is the single most important factor in the immediate management of head injuries.

- Features which may be peculiar to the airway care of head trauma include:
  - Impacted facial fractures obstructing the pharynx require reduction by manually lifting the fragment anteriorly.
  - If endotracheal intubation is required before x-rays of the cervical spine have been performed, the possibility of cervical spine injury should be remembered and movement of the neck reduced to an absolute minimum.
- Associated chest injuries merit rapid treatment.
- Throughout the examination and management of the patient, oxygen should be administered in as high a concentration as possible.
- Arterial blood gases should be taken as soon as practicable and repeated when airway control and ventilation are stabilized.
- In patients requiring assisted ventilation, hyperventilation (to reduce Pa_{CO_2} to 3–4 kPa) may be of value in reducing raised intracranial pressure.
- Pass a nasogastric tube and empty the stomach to reduce the possibility of aspiration and prevent gastric dilatation.

Shock
- Features of shock are rarely related to head injury alone. In a shocked patient with a head injury and no

overt site(s) of blood loss, intra-abdominal or intra-thoracic blood loss should be considered.
- Rarely, shock can result due to bleeding from large scalp lacerations or if a large scalp artery has been involved. Brisk aural haemorrhage may result from damage to the carotid artery in the base of skull.
- All serious head injuries require an i.v. line *in situ*. In the absence of hypovolaemia infuse 0.9% saline slowly.
- Send blood sample for grouping and cross-matching.

Fitting
- Following head injury, fitting may result from increasing intracranial pressure or focal lesion(s), e.g. intracranial bleeding, depressed skull fracture.
- Fitting will cause a secondary deterioration due to respiratory embarrassment and a further rise in intracranial pressure.
- Should be treated with i.v. diazepam, titrated to control the fitting (usual dosage required 5–20 mg).

Neurological deterioration
- Inadequacy of ventilation and/or circulating blood volume deficits must always be excluded before any deterioration in consciousness is considered to be due to an intracranial lesion alone.
- Thereafter, any deterioration in consciousness (i.e. a

numerical fall on the Glasgow coma scale) is suggestive of intracranial pathology.

- The use of an agent to lower intracranial pressure may be contemplated in such patients. These agents should not be given indiscriminately since rebound increases in intracranial pressure can occur, or haematomata may be encouraged to enlarge further. Wherever possible the situation should be discussed with a neurosurgical specialist prior to administration.
- Suitable agents for lowering intracranial pressure are:
  - Mannitol: 0.5–2 mg/kg i.v. infused over 20–30 minutes.
  - Frusemide: 20–40 mg i.v.

SPINAL INJURY

GENERAL POINTS

- Suspect spinal injury in all patients with neck pain after trauma, all head injuries, and patients with multiple injuries.
- During the initial resuscitation and examination of the patient, head and neck movements should be prevented either by manual control or the application of a cervical collar.
- When transferring the patient to a trolley or bed,

alignment of the spinal column must be maintained (this requires four people, one of whom maintains cervical traction and head control during the procedure).
- The prompt correction of hypovolaemia and hypoxia is essential to prevent further cord damage.
- The levels at which spinal injury most frequently occurs are C_{1-2}, C_7-T_1, $T_{12}-L_1$ and L_{4-5}.

HISTORY

- An account of the following features should be obtained from the patient and/or attendant:
  - Limb movements and/or weakness after injury.
  - Headache, neck pain, paraesthesiae.

Note: a patient with occipital headache and/or supporting his head in his hands may have an odontoid fracture.

EXAMINATION

- Carefully remove all the patient's clothing to allow a full neurological examination.
- Note any evidence of the mechanism(s) involved in the injury, e.g. injury to chin indicating a hyperextension injury.
- Roll the patient (see above) to allow examination of

the spine for deformity, tenderness, gaps or boggy
areas in the interspinous ligament.
- In an unconscious patient record the presence/absence
and symmetry of limb movement spontaneously, and
in response to painful stimuli.
- In conscious patients record power in each limb and
muscle group.
- Remember that limb weakness may also be due to a
hemiplegia or brachial plexus injury.
- Examine reflexes. Note that the motor root values *at
cord level* are:

	Cord level
Biceps jerk	$C_{5-(6)}$
Supinator jerk	$C_{(5)-6}$
Triceps jerk	C_{6-7}
Knee jerk	L_{3-4}
Ankle jerk	L_5-S_1
Upper abdominal reflexes	T_{7-9}
Lower abdominal reflexes	T_{10-12}

- Carefully assess any sensory deficit; test for light-
touch and pinprick sensation, taking particular care to
test the saddle area and perineum.
- Note that persistent penile erection may indicate major
cord damage.

INVESTIGATIONS

X-ray

General points
- Good quality radiographic films are essential.
- Standard anteroposterior and lateral views are always required. Other projections which may be indicated include:
  - Open-mouth view of odontoid peg.
  - Oblique or lateral views in flexion or extension.
  - 'Swimmer's view' of the lower cervical/upper thoracic region.

  If doubt exists as to stability of the injured spine, the taking of such radiographs should be supervised by a senior doctor.
- It is important to obtain a full-length view of the cervical spine from C_1–T_1, if necessary by using longitudinal arm traction.
- Disruption of the anterior or posterior longitudinal spinal ligaments may merely result in small flake fractures or even no radiological abnormality in the neutral position. Soft tissue swelling related to the spinal vertebrae may suggest the presence of this type of injury which will render the spine potentially unstable. Supervised flexion/extension views may be required for diagnosis.

●The interpretation of spinal radiographs can be extremely difficult. Specialist advice should be sought if any doubt exists.

MANAGEMENT

Cervical spine injuries

●Injuries resulting in high cord lesions (C_{1-4}) usually cause apnoea; such patients will require immediate assisted ventilation.

●Respiratory embarrassment may result from cervical and upper thoracic cord lesions *per se*, or as a consequence of associated soft tissue injury.

●Vasomotor disturbances, bradycardias, hypotension, and hypothermia may occur due to reflex peripheral vasodilatation.

●Hyperextension injuries are especially common in the elderly and in patients with cervical spondylosis. These injuries are usually stable, but central cord damage (affecting upper limbs more than lower limbs) may occur.

●In patients who are self-ventilating, administer a high concentration (40–60%) of inspired oxygen via face mask. Check arterial blood gases and seek specialist help.

●If endotracheal intubation is required before specialist

help can be obtained (e.g. in an apnoeic patient or one with severe respiratory embarrassment), neck movement during the procedure must be kept to an absolute minimum (see page 29).

- In flexion injuries with or without displacement, apply a temporary cervical collar. If further procedures (e.g. laparotomy or delays in transfer) are anticipated, apply skull traction (e.g. using Gardner–Wells skull calipers applied 5 cm above the external acoustic meatus initially applying 5–10 lb of traction).

Thoracic and lumbar spine injuries

- Stable wedge compression fractures are the commonest type of injury. They require specialist referral for bed rest and analgesia.
- Unstable fracture/dislocations are usually the result of major trauma and associated cord damage is often severe.
- Unstable thoracic spine injuries may have associated mediastinal injury, the management of which will take priority.
- Lumbar spine injuries may be associated with hypovolaemic shock as a consequence of local blood loss and retroperitoneal haematomata. Associated renal, ureteric and intra-abdominal injuries are also common (see page 71).

60

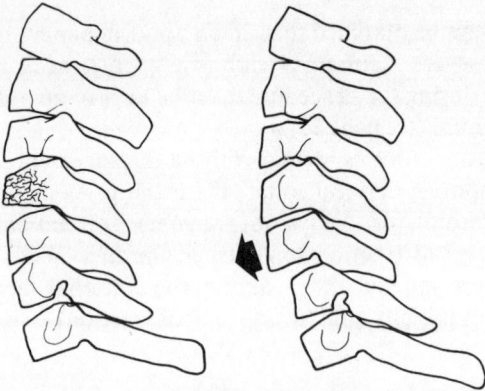

Fig. 14. Stable (left) and unstable (right) spinal injuries

CHEST INJURY

GENERAL POINTS

- Serious injury to the chest is commonly under-estimated.
- The consequent hypoxia and blood loss, if unrecognized, will compound the effects of other injuries.

HISTORY

- Obtain a good account of the accident. A description of the wreckage (including speeds involved) and the mechanism of the chest injury will lead to an accurate presumptive diagnosis.

- Pain:
  - Localized (? minor rib injury).
  - 'Back pain' (? major rib injury and/or mediastinal damage).
  - 'Chest tightness" (? mediastinal injury or pneumothorax).
  - 'Shoulder pain' (? referred from neck or subdiaphragmatic pathology).
- Is dyspnoea:
  - Due to pain?
  - Related to stridor?
  - 'Just cannot get breath' (? pneumothorax, haemothorax).
- Any past history of chronic chest disease.

EXAMINATION

- Do not examine the chest in isolation.
- Inspection. Look specifically for:
  - Colour of skin.
  - Dyspnoea.
  - Stridor.
  - 'Grunting' during respiration.
  - Distension of neck veins.
  - Obvious injury/bruising/imprinting.
  - Symmetrical movement/flail segments.

62

- Palpation:
  - Tracheal position/deviation.
  - Surgical emphysema.
  - Tenderness.
  - Crepitus.
  - Praecordial thrills.
  - Peripheral pulses.
- Auscultation:
  - Breath sounds.
  - Added sounds—crepitation, crepitus, 'click' of pneumothorax (usually left-sided and synchronous with systole).
  - Heart sounds, murmurs.
- Percussion (if possible).

INVESTIGATIONS

No investigation should delay urgent treatment.

Radiography

Chest x-ray
- If at all possible, the chest x-ray should be performed with the patient erect, as in supine films, pneumo- or haemothoraces may be easily missed (Fig. 15), and the mediastinum will appear falsely widened.
- If a pneumothorax is suspected a radiograph in expiration should also be performed.

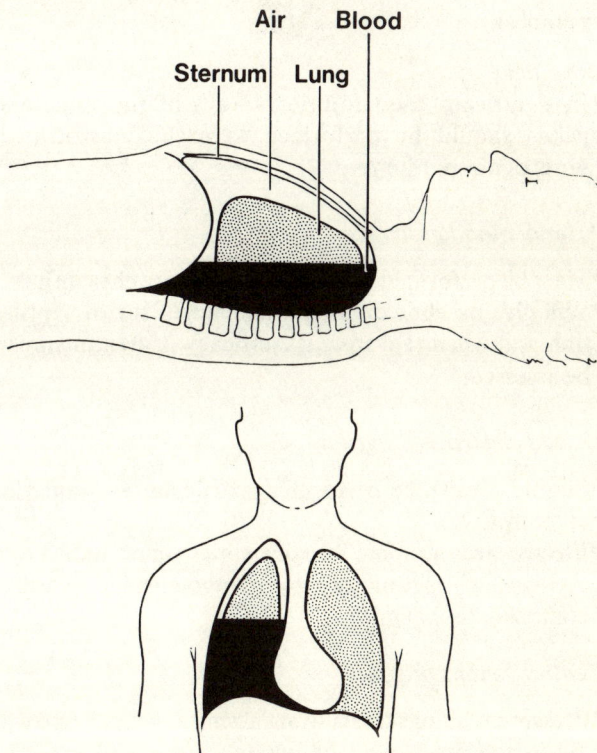

Fig. 15. Diagram illustrating how pneumo- and haemo-thoraces are more obvious when radiographs are taken in the erect position

- Serial films may assist in monitoring any developing pathology.

Other films
- In significant chest injuries, x-rays of the spine and pelvis should be performed to exclude associated, unrecognized injury.

Arterial blood gases

- Must be performed in moderate or severe chest injury.
- Will give baseline data regarding adequacy of ventilation and when repeated, the efficacy of treatment can be assessed.

12 lead electrocardiogram

- Should always be performed, particularly in anterior chest injury.
- Electrocardiographic abnormalities may indicate a myocardial aetiology for hypotension (cardiac contusion/ischaemia).

Central venous pressure

- Pressure readings taken using a central venous line will aid in the assessment of hypovolaemia and assist in monitoring i.v. replacement therapy.
- May help to exclude cardiac tamponade.

PENETRATING CHEST TRAUMA

General points

- Do not probe chest wounds.
- If a foreign body is still present, leave it undisturbed *in situ*.
- A chest drain must be inserted on the side of the penetrating injury and should be introduced outwith the wound, by a separate incision (see page 158).
- Remember that injury may have occurred to organs in the chest or abdomen apparently remote from the surface site of injury.
- The possibility of cardiac tamponade and/or mediastinal damage must always be considered (see page 69).
- Large sucking chest wounds should be covered with a dry sterile dressing; after chest drain(s) has been inserted, the patient is managed as for blunt chest injury (see below).

BLUNT CHEST TRAUMA: SUMMARY OF INDIVIDUAL INJURIES

'Simple' rib fracture

- Associated pain is localized, aggravated by respiration or on springing the chest.

- Remember that costal cartilage fractures are not apparent radiographically.
- 'Simple' rib fractures are usually of little significance, apart from the patient's requirement for analgesia. However, a patient with more than two rib fractures merits specialist referral for admission and observation.
- Fractures of the clavicle and first or second ribs implies a severe chest injury with possible damage to subclavian vessels or other injury, e.g. to head and neck. Specialist advice should be sought.
- A single rib fracture in a patient with chronic airways disease may require admission.

Sternal fracture

- Is clinically detected by local tenderness and if displaced, as a palpable 'step'.
- A lateral sternal x-ray view should be performed.
- In younger patients in whom displacement at the fracture site is greater than the anteroposterior width of the sternum on x-ray, or any sternal fracture in an elderly patient, refer for specialist advice and consider the possibility of associated mediastinal and/or myocardial damage.

Flail chest

- Summon experienced help early as therapy will be required urgently.

- The diagnosis is a clinical one, paradoxical chest wall movement occurring with respiration.
- In a patient with rapid, shallow respiration it may be easier to detect paradoxical movement by gentle palpation rather than observation.
- Give a high concentration (40–60%) of inspired oxygen and check arterial blood gases on presentation and when the patient's condition is stable.
- Analgesia: inhaled nitrous oxide/oxygen or i.v. morphine cautiously titrated to the patient's response should be given if required.
- Treat any associated pneumothorax or haemothorax promptly (see below).
- If the patient is 'in extremis', immediate endotracheal intubation and positive pressure ventilation will be required.
- In patients who are being ventilated, consider inserting bilateral chest drains prophylactically to prevent the possibility of a developing tension pneumothorax.

Pneumothorax

- The diagnosis of pneumothorax related to trauma can be difficult.
- Remember that on a supine chest x-ray, pneumothoraces may not be apparent (see Fig. 15).
- Palpate for subcutaneous emphysema over chest and neck.

●Early drainage of the pneumothorax using an intercostal catheter (see page 158) is required.

Tension pneumothorax

●The patient will exhibit increasing dyspnoea and
distress with ipsilateral reduced air entry and breath
sounds and tracheal deviation to opposite side.
●If the presence of a pneumothorax under 'tension' is
suspected, a large bore cannula (e.g. 12–14G) should
be immediately inserted into the second intercostal
space in the mid-clavicular line to decompress the
'tension' and 'buy time' while a standard chest drain is
inserted.
●Tension pneumothoraces are liable to develop very
rapidly in patients being ventilated with positive
pressure.

Haemothorax

●The patient will present with signs of a chest injury and
developing hypovolaemia.
●An associated ipsilateral pneumothorax is common
and will require appropriate treatment.
●The rate of volume replacement should be guided by
the clinical response to i.v. fluids and *not* to the
apparent blood loss from intercostal drains.

Aortic or mediastinal vessel rupture

• A history of rapid deceleration injury is common.
• A sternal fracture, anterior flail chest, unexplained hypo- or hypertension, murmurs or discrepancy between brachial and femoral pulses may be present.
• On an erect anteroposterior chest x-ray, widening of the upper mediastinum may be seen. (If possible, serial radiographs should be performed.)
• Following initial resuscitation, such patients must be urgently referred for angiography and/or thoracotomy.

Cardiac tamponade

• May occur as a result of blunt or penetrating chest trauma.
• Restlessness, hypotension, increasing dyspnoea, differential cyanosis, pulsus paradoxus, and distended neck veins are frequently present.
• The response to i.v. fluid therapy may suggest the presence of tamponade; a rising central venous pressure (usually in excess of $20\,cmH_2O$) without improvement in pulse and blood pressure is strongly suggestive of developing tamponade.
• On chest x-ray, an enlarged globular heart may be seen, but the heart size is more often normal as the pericardium is a relatively stiff, inflexible sac.

- Urgent aspiration and specialist referral is indicated (see page 162).

Ruptured diaphragm

- May be caused by blunt injury to the abdomen or pelvis and is more commonly left-sided.
- Dyspnoea is aggravated by the supine position and occasionally bowel sounds are audible in the chest.
- Urgent treatment is usually related to any associated (haemo-) pneumothorax.
- Consider the possibility of related splenic, hepatic, or pelvic injuries.

Ruptured trachea

- This injury is very rare and usually presents with bruising and surgical emphysema in the neck together with stridor, severe dyspnoea, and cyanosis.
- Seek urgent specialist help; maintain on supportive therapy with a high concentration (40–60%) of inspired oxygen and avoid attempts at endotracheal intubation if the patient's clinical state permits.

ABDOMINAL INJURY

GENERAL POINTS

- The diagnosis of abdominal injury is often difficult.
- Intraperitoneal bleeding is often only suspected when other injuries which may cause hypovolaemia have been excluded.
- Remember that trauma to the chest, spine, pelvis, perineum, and thighs may involve intra-abdominal injury and vice versa.

HISTORY

- The nature of the accident, the forces exerted and any element of crushing are helpful in assessing the possibility of intra-abdominal injury.
- Ask attendants if:
  - The patient has complained of pain.
  - The patient's condition has deteriorated.
  - The patient has passed urine since the accident.
- Ask the patient specifically about:
  - Pain—site, radiation, type.
  - Shoulder pain—may imply referred pain from diaphragm.
  - Chest pain, or pain on respiration.

EXAMINATION

- Continuous observation of the patient's vital signs and repeated clinical examination are mandatory.
- General:
  - Skin colour, sweating, and peripheral perfusion.
  - Conscious level.
- Specific:
  - Movement of abdominal wall with respiration.
  - Obvious or penetrating injury.
  - Bruising or imprinted pattern of clothing ('imprinting' strongly suggests rupture or major injury to intra-abdominal organs).
  - Swelling/distension.
  - Blood at the external urethral meatus, vagina, anus.
  - Rectal examination.
- Palpate for local tenderness or discomfort on 'springing' of the chest and pelvis.
  Note: signs of guarding and rebound are difficult to interpret in the context of abdominal trauma and auscultation and abdominal girth measurements are similarly of little diagnostic help.

INVESTIGATIONS

- Continuously monitor:
  - Pulse.

- •Blood pressure.
- •Central venous pressure (in serious injury).
- •Test urine for blood (by catheter if necessary—except if the possibility of urethral injury exists, when urethral catheterization is contraindicated).
- •X-ray:
  - •Chest: look for rib fractures (which may suggest injury to underlying organs), (haemo-) pneumo-thorax, free gas under the diaphragm, and abnormal diaphragmatic contours.
  - •Pelvis: remember that any pelvic fracture is likely to be associated with 1–4 litres of blood loss. Fractures of the ischial and pubic rami are particularly prone to have associated urethral and/or bladder injury.
  - •Plain abdominal film: look for the renal outlines, psoas shadows, fractures of transverse processes may accompany associated ureteric or renal trauma or retroperitoneal haemorrhage), and free intra-peritoneal gas.
- •Intravenous urograms, urethrograms, and angiography may be indicated following the initial assessment, management, and specialist referral.
- •Peritoneal lavage (see page 165): is indicated in the following situations to assess the presence of intra-peritoneal bleeding:
  - •Patients with multiple injuries (particularly if associated with altered consciousness).

•Patients with an abdominal injury and 'unexplained' hypotension.

MANAGEMENT
•Send blood sample for grouping and cross-matching.
•Insert an i.v. cannula and commence volume replacement as appropriate (see page 34).
•Give a high concentration of inspired oxygen via face mask.
•Treat other possible causes of hypotension, e.g. associated chest injury, inadequately splinted fractures.
•Analgesia: give i.v. morphine titrated against response *after* the patient has been fully examined and assessed.
•Pass a nasogastric tube and aspirate stomach contents.
•The Newcastle G-suit/military anti-shock trousers: the application of these devices may be useful in severe lower abdominal trauma. Remember that once applied further abdominal examination is impossible and the patient is committed to urgent laparotomy (see page 37).

SUMMARY OF INDIVIDUAL INJURIES

Penetrating abdominal trauma
•There is usually little difficulty in diagnosis. Entry and exit wounds may indicate which organs are likely to have been involved.

- Do not probe tracks.
- 'Open' abdominal wall injuries should have warm saline soaks applied to exposed tissues, otherwise injuries should be treated as below.
- All penetrating wounds must be referred for a specialist surgical opinion.

Blunt abdominal trauma

Liver, spleen, and mesenteric injuries
- Individual organ injuries may have little difference in their clinical picture and the features of hypovolaemia are usually the most apparent abnormality.
- The areas of injury, tenderness, and guarding in the early stages may be of value in determining which specific organs have been damaged.

Urinary tract injuries
- Loin pain/tenderness in association with haematuria indicates renal trauma.
- Associated ureteric injuries are uncommon and in such cases haematuria is not *invariably* present, e.g. complete ureteric transection.
- Any haematuria following trauma is an indication for an intravenous urogram, the timing of which depends upon the severity of haematuria and associated injuries.

- Injury to the bladder may present with features of a perforated intraperitoneal viscus or with extra-peritoneal extravasation. Commonly there is an associated pelvic ring fracture, bruising around the perineum and blood at the external urethral meatus. In such cases do *not* attempt to pass a urethral catheter.

Retroperitoneal trauma

- The diagnosis of retroperitoneal trauma and haemorrhage can only be *suspected* in the emergency situation, as there are no specific pathognomonic features.
- A high index of suspicion should, however, be maintained in hypovolaemic traumatized patients in whom there is no overt blood loss and no detectable haemothorax or haemoperitoneum.
- On plain abdominal x-ray, the psoas shadows may be indistinct and fractures of the transverse spinal processes may be present.
- Peritoneal lavage, if performed, may be weakly positive or negative.

THE BURNED PATIENT

HISTORY

About the fire

- What was burning (e.g. furniture, fabrics, polystyrene foam)?

- Was it an enclosed space?
- Was there an explosion?
- For how long was patient exposed to fire or smoke?
- Note the time elapsed from injury/exposure to presentation in hospital.

About the patient

- Past medical history, with particular reference to chronic chest pathology and ischaemic heart disease.
- Current medications.
- Precipitating cause(s) for exposure to hazard, e.g. alcohol or drug use, hypoglycaemia, epilepsy, cerebro-vascular accident, trauma, etc.

EXAMINATION

Repiratory

- Look for burns of face or neck, singeing of hair, hoarseness, oropharyngeal oedema, and sooty particles in pharynx or below vocal cords.
- Auscultate chest for signs of bronchospasm and atelectasis.
- Ensure that full thickness burns of chest wall are not restricting respiratory movements.
- Check peak expiratory flow rate if possible.

Extent of burns

●The extent of burned body surface is much more important in the initial management than the depth of the burn.
●For adults, the 'rule of nines' can be used (Fig. 16):

Head	9%
Trunk	18% front
	18% back
Arms	9% each
Legs	18% each

●Alternatively the area of patient's outstretched hand (approximately 1%) can be used to estimate area involved.
●Although electrical burns may have small areas of skin damage, they are invariably full thickness. Entrance and exit wounds should be looked for. There may be associated musculoskeletal or cardiac injury.

Cardiovascular

●Signs of 'shock' (see page 33) may be present due to hypovolaemia and aggravated by the effects of smoke inhalation on cardiac and respiratory function.
●Remember that peripheral circulation may be impaired due to 'tourniquet-effect' of circumferential burns.

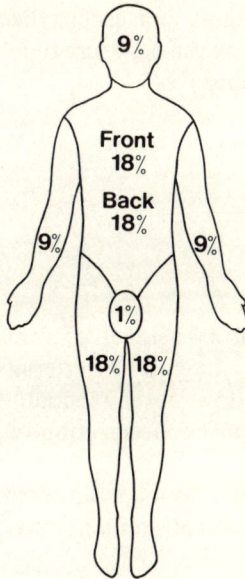

Fig. 16. The rule of 'nines'

INVESTIGATIONS

In burns involving more than 10% of body surface, electrical burns, and in all cases of suspected smoke inhalation, the following investigations should be performed:

- Arterial blood gases and carboxyhaemoglobin level. (Note the time between exposure to inhalational injury and blood sampling.)
- Chest x-ray.
- Electrocardiogram.

MANAGEMENT

Respiratory

- Frequent clinical assessment of respiratory function together with measurement of arterial blood gases and peak expiratory flow rate is essential.
- Give high (40–60%) concentration of inspired oxygen via face mask.
- If patient is unable to maintain airway, endotracheal intubation and assisted ventilation will be required.

Cardiovascular

- Greater than 15% burned skin surface (or greater than 10% in elderly patients) will require i.v. fluid replacement and cardiac monitoring.
- The insertion of i.v. cannulae should, if possible, be away from burned skin.
- In shocked patients, a central venous line will aid monitoring of cardiovascular status and volume replacement.

- Send blood sample for grouping and cross-matching.
- Volume replacement: give 0.9% saline or Ringer's lactate solution. Over the initial 4–6 hours since injury, requirements may be roughly estimated according to the formula:

$$\frac{\text{Volume required}}{\text{(ml)}} = \frac{\text{Percentage area}}{\text{of burn}} \times \frac{\text{Body weight}}{\text{(kg)}}$$

- In burned patients requiring volume replacement, insert a urinary catheter to assess urine output and test urine for blood and myoglobin.

General

- Analgesia: i.v. morphine, titrated against the clinical response, is the most effective and rapid form of analgesia.
- After examination of the burn, cover with a clean sheet until patient is transferred for further care.
- If full thickness burns of the trunk are causing reduction of chest wall movement and resultant respiratory embarrassment, incise using a sterile technique. Similar treatment is required for the limbs if there is a 'tourniquet-effect' causing impaired circulation. These incisions should be longitudinal and of sufficient depth to relieve the constricting effect.

Section 3

ACUTE CHEST PAIN

COMMON CAUSES OF CHEST PAIN

Central	*Lateralized*
Myocardial ischaemia/infarction	Rib fracture(s)
Oesophageal causes, e.g.	Pneumothorax
oesophageal reflex, hiatus hernia	Pneumonia
Pericarditis	Pulmonary
Dissecting aortic aneurysm	infarction
Major pulmonary embolus	Viral myositis/
Perforated intra-abdominal viscus	costochondritis
	Herpes zoster

HISTORY

• Ask the patient about the following features of the pain:
  • Site (central, lateralized).
  • Onset, duration, character, and radiation.
  • Relieving or aggravating factors, e.g. position, respiration, exertion, administration of glyceryl trinitrate or antacids.
• Associated symptoms:
  • Nausea, vomiting, sweating.
  • Dyspnoea.
  • Palpitations.

●Past history:
  ·Previous episodes.
  ·Recent chest, spinal or abdominal trauma.
  ·Hypertension, ischaemic heart disease, obstructive airways disease, dyspeptic symptoms.
●Current drug therapy.

EXAMINATION

General

●Mood of patient.
●Skin colour (pallor, cyanosis), sweating, rashes, and peripheral perfusion.
●Localized tenderness, pain on springing chest.

Cardiovascular system

●Pulse rate, rhythm, and volume. Check carotid and femoral pulses and their synchronicity.
●Blood pressure (check in *both* arms).
●Heart sounds (murmurs, extra sounds, friction rubs).
●Jugular venous pressure.
●Bruits.

Respiratory system

●Is dyspnoea or tachypnoea present?
●Position of trachea.

●Percussion note.
●Auscultation.

INVESTIGATIONS

●12 lead electrocardiogram:
  ·Look specifically for:
    ·Rhythm abnormalities.
    ·Changes of acute infarction, ischaemia, or peri-carditis.
    ·Changes suggesting acute right heart strain.
●Chest x-ray:
  ·Look specifically for:
    ·Pneumothorax (both inspiratory and expiratory films are required).
    ·Rib fractures (lateral/oblique films may be indicated).
    ·Cardiomegaly or abnormal cardiac contour.
    ·Gas under diaphragm(s).
●Arterial blood gases.

MYOCARDIAL ISCHAEMIA/INFARCTION

Clinical features

●'Crushing' or 'tight' retrosternal chest pain, usually unrelieved by posture, respiration, antacids, or rest.

88

- Glyceryl trinitrate may relieve the pain associated with myocardial ischaemia (and occasionally oesophageal pain) but will rarely do so completely in the case of myocardial infarction.
- Pain may be present in the arms, jaw, neck, or the back, with or without retrosternal chest pain.
- A past history of ischaemic heart disease, hypertension, or diabetes may be elicited.
- Drugs: is the patient taking β-blockers, anti-anginal drugs, antihypertensive agents or diuretics?
- The clinical state may vary from that of a fully conscious patient with a mild chest discomfort, to that of an obtunded patient in cardiogenic shock.
- Sweating, nausea, dyspnoea, and angor animi are commonly present.
- Look for evidence of acute cardiac failure, viz. fine persistent crepitations on chest auscultation, added heart sounds, jugular venous pressure.

Investigations

- Electrocardiogram: ST–T wave abnormalities (convex upward ST elevation, T wave inversion) are the commonest *early* changes (see Fig. 17). If pathological Q waves develop this usually occurs some hours/days following infarction. Note, however, that a normal electrocardiogram does *not* exclude the possibility of acute infarction or ischaemia.

89

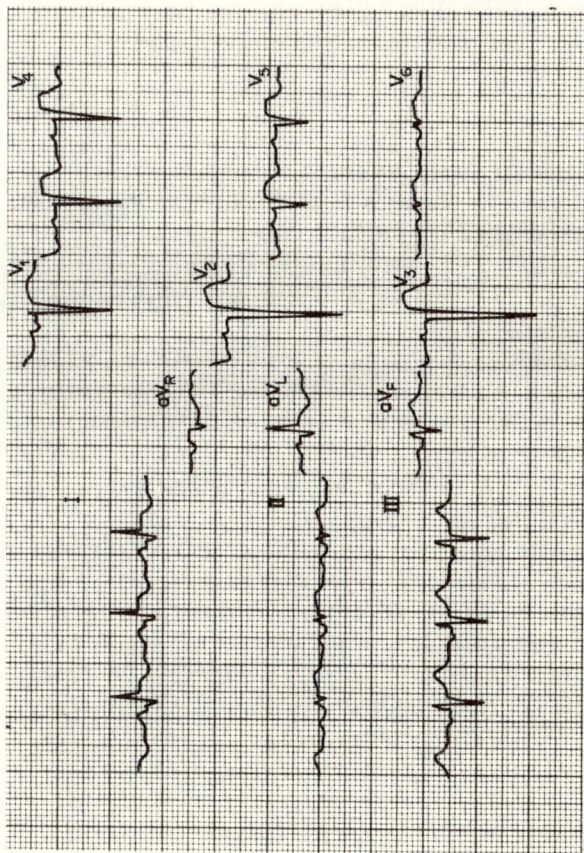

Fig. 17

●Chest x-ray: look specifically for signs of cardiac failure (see page 108) and/or cardiomegaly.

Management

●Attach the patient to a cardiac monitor.
●Insert an i.v. cannula flushed with heparinized saline and occluded.
●If required, give i.v. morphine (dosage required is usually 5–15 mg) for analgesia and relief of psychic distress.
●Administer a high concentration (40–60%) of inspired oxygen. If the patient has evidence, or a past history of obstructive airways disease, give 28–30% concentration of inspired oxygen via face mask and check arterial blood gases 15–20 minutes after commencing oxygen therapy.
●If signs of left ventricular failure are present, give a short acting 'loop' diuretic (e.g. frusemide) by i.v. route. The dose will depend upon the severity of the left ventricular failure and whether or not the patient regularly takes diuretics, but is commonly 20–120 mg.
●Refer for specialist care.

Note

●Patients with an increasing frequency or severity of

anginal attacks (crescendo angina) require specialist referral.
- Arrhythmias can be provoked in any patient as a consequence of sympathetic overactivity; therefore the patient must be constantly reassured, given adequate analgesia, transportation should be smooth, and iatrogenic insults reduced to a minimum.
- Ischaemic heart disease can present at any age. Do not ignore a history suggestive of myocardial ischaemia in a young patient on the grounds of age alone.

ACUTE PERICARDITIS

Clinical features

- Midsternal discomfort, aggravated by movement and respiration, is a common complaint.
- A past history of recent viral illness, myocardial infarction, connective tissue disorder, trauma, or uraemia may be obtained.
- Listen for pericardial friction rubs by auscultating with the patient in different positions and phases of respiration.
- Look for signs suggesting (a large) pericardial effusion —dyspnoea, soft heart sounds, pulsus paradoxus, Küssmaul's sign (jugular venous pressure *rises* with inspiration).

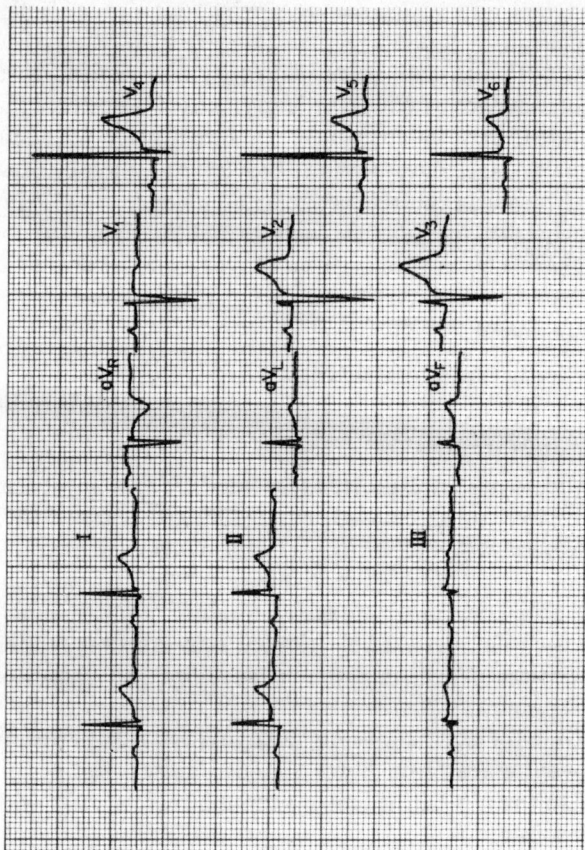

Fig. 18

Investigations

- Electrocardiogram: commonly, widespread concave upwards ST segment elevation is present (see Fig. 18).
- Chest x-ray: note that the heart size is usually normal (even when a large pericardial effusion is present).

Management

- Refer for inpatient care. (Acute treatment is rarely required.)

AORTIC DISSECTION

Clinical features

- A history of 'tearing' or 'ripping', retrosternal or epigastric pain of sudden onset which may radiate to back or neck (but rarely to arms) may be elicited.
- The patient may present as a 'collapse', with altered consciousness or with signs of a mono-, di- or paraplegia.
- Ask specifically regarding a past history of hypertension or recent chest injury (see page 60).
- Look for:
  - Features of shock (see page 38).
  - Signs of differential perfusion or cyanosis.

•Pulse abnormalities and inequalities (measure blood pressure in both arms).
•Bruits (neck, chest, abdomen).

Investigations

●Chest x-ray: appearances may be normal or show mediastinal widening, pleural effusions, or aortic calcification.
●Electrocardiogram: commonly non-specific ST–T wave changes are present. Rarely, if the dissection has tracked proximally to involve the aortic root, 'classical' changes of acute myocardial ischaemia or infarction can be seen.

Management

●Attach patient to a cardiac monitor.
●Insert i.v. cannula, take and send a suitable blood sample for grouping and cross-matching.
●Administer a high concentration (40–60%) of inspired oxygen via face mask.
●Analgesia: give i.v. morphine—titrate dose given against clinical response (usual dose 5–15 mg).
●Insert a urinary catheter.
●Refer for specialist advice regarding the requirement for emergency angiography and surgery.

MAJOR PULMONARY EMBOLISM (see page 111)

LATERALIZED CHEST PAIN

In general, lateralized chest pain is rarely due to a life-threatening process. The aetiology is usually rapidly apparent from clinical examination and/or chest x-ray and the common causes are listed above. In particular examine the patient for:
- Areas of localized rib or intercostal tenderness.
- Discomfort on springing the chest.
- Inequalities or abnormalities in percussion note or breath sounds.
- Skin rashes.
- Signs of deep venous thrombosis.

ACUTE DYSPNOEA

COMMON CAUSES

- Asthma.
- Acute exacerbation of chronic bronchitis.
- Pulmonary oedema.
- Pneumonia/acute bronchitis.
- Pneumothorax.
- Pulmonary thromboembolism.

LESS COMMON CAUSES

- Psychogenic dyspnoea ('hysterical hyperventilation').
- Acute metabolic acidosis.
- Pleural effusion.
- Inhaled foreign body.
- Carcinoma of bronchus.

HISTORY

- Rate of onset.
- Associated symptoms:
  - Orthopnoea.
  - Wheeze.
  - Chest pain.
  - Cough, sputum, haemoptysis.
- Previous similar episodes.
- Ingestion of drugs.
- Renal disease/diabetes.

EXAMINATION

General

- Conscious level.
- Cyanosis.
- Peripheral perfusion/sweating.

- Evidence of anaemia or polycythaemia.
- Fever.
- Finger clubbing.
- Evidence of diabetes or renal failure.

Cardiovascular

- Pulse rate, rhythm, and volume (? presence of arrhythmia, pulsus paradoxus, or pulsus alternans).
- Added heart sounds/murmurs.
- Blood pressure.

Respiratory

- Ventilatory rate and pattern (shallow/gasping/periodic).
- Chest symmetry, intercostal indrawing.
- Position of trachea and apex beat.
- Percussion note.
- Air entry, bronchial breathing, and added sounds (crepitations/rhonchi).

Note:

In auscultation of the chest:
- Comparative assessment of air entry noise in both sides of the chest is important.
- Auscultatory findings should always be taken in context with the rest of examination.

•The interpretation of auscultatory findings can be difficult. There is no substitute for a good quality chest x-ray.

INVESTIGATIONS

Chest x-ray

Look for signs of:
•Consolidation (lobar/lobular/patchy).
•Pneumothorax. Whenever possible, erect inspiratory and expiratory films should be performed.
•Pleural effusion(s).
•Pulmonary oedema:
  ·Cardiomegaly.
  ·Enlarged hilar vessels.
  ·Increased vascularity (especially increased diameter of upper lobe vessels).
  ·Septal lines (Kerley's 'B' lines), fluid in horizontal fissure. 'Ground glass' appearance of interstitial fluid.
•Chronic bronchitis and emphysema:
  ·There may be *no* abnormality.
  ·Hyperinflated lung fields, a long narrow mediastinum, flat diaphragms, prominent pulmonary arteries and bullae may be seen in advanced chronic bronchitis and emphysema.

Arterial blood gases

- Arterial blood gas analysis is essential in all dyspnoeic or cyanosed patients.
- Ideally the sample should be taken with the patient breathing air prior to starting oxygen therapy.

Electrocardiogram

- May be of value in the investigation of pulmonary oedema, metabolic acidosis, pulmonary thromboembolism, and advanced airways disease.

ACUTE SEVERE ASTHMA

Any asthmatic patient whose symptoms have failed to respond to their regular bronchodilator therapy has acute severe asthma.

Clinical history (if possible)

- Length of history and mode of onset of this attack.
- Previous severe attacks, hospitalization, mechanical ventilation.
- What usually gets the attack better? Response to steroids?
- Recent drug intake, e.g. salicylates.

Clinical assessment

- Audible wheeze is *not* a good index of severity.
- The peak expiratory flow rate should be measured.
- The patient should be regarded as seriously ill if there is:
  - Disturbed conscious level.
  - Exhaustion and/or dehydration.
  - Inability to talk due to dyspnoea.
  - Central cyanosis.
  - Tachycardia greater than 120/min.
  - Palpable pulsus paradoxus.
  - A peak expiratory flow rate less than 100 l/min.

Investigations

Chest x-ray
Look specifically for:
- Pneumothorax.
- Pneumomediastinum.
- Rib fractures.

Arterial blood gases
- Most cases show a slight reduction in PaO_2 with a reduced (or at lower limit of normal) $PaCO_2$ due to hyperventilation.
- A normal $PaCO_2$ in the presence of hypoxia may *not* be a favourable sign and should be checked later.

- A raised $Pa\text{CO}_2$ is ominous and may indicate a need for mechanical ventilation. It should be checked within 30 minutes of institution of therapy or sooner if there is a change in clinical condition.

Management

General points
- Do not leave a severe asthmatic unobserved— deterioration may occur very quickly and the patient may not be able to call for help.
- Anaesthetic and medical specialists should be informed early.
- *Never sedate* an agitated distressed asthmatic. The combination of severe asthma and sedation may be fatal.
- Give a high concentration (40–60%) of inspired oxygen via face mask after taking arterial blood gases.
- Insert an i.v. cannula. A slow infusion of 0.9% saline should be commenced if the patient has signs of salt and water depletion.

Drug therapy

β-Adrenergic stimulants
- These should preferably be given by inhalation as the resultant bronchodilation persists longer and has fewer side effects than after i.v. administration.

- The cheapest and simplest way is in nebulized form, e.g. Wright's nebulizer driven by high flow oxygen.
- There is no evidence that administration by intermittent positive pressure ventilation is more effective.
- *Dosages:*
  - Salbutamol: 2.5–5 mg of respirator solution in 5 ml saline.
  - Terbutaline: 5 mg of respirator solution in 5 ml saline.
  - If a nebulizer is not available, give salbutamol by i.v. infusion (dose: 0.25 mg over 5 minutes).

Aminophylline

- Although a very effective bronchodilator, this drug is potentially dangerous especially in hypoxic, severely ill patients.
- It is probably no longer a first-line drug since the introduction of β-adrenergic stimulants.
- The therapeutic ratio is narrow and ideally treatment should be monitored by plasma theophylline levels.
- Dose: 6 mg/kg i.v. given over 30 minutes followed by 0.5 mg/kg as an infusion.
- The dosage requirement may be considerably less in elderly patients, patients with liver dysfunction, cardiac failure, or those already taking oral theophyllines.

Steroids

- Give i.v. corticosteroids as early as possible. The initial management period of a severe attack often means 'tiding the patient over' with bronchodilators until systemic corticosteroids take effect in 30–90 minutes.

● *Dosage:* hydrocortisone 4 mg/kg as an i.v. bolus.

Artificial ventilation

The overall clinical situation should be continuously reviewed and artificial ventilation seriously considered if:

● The patient is clinically exhausted with rising pulse rate and inability to clear secretions.

● There is a rising $Pa\text{CO}_2$ despite institution of the above therapy.

ACUTE EXACERBATION OF CHRONIC BRONCHITIS

General points

● The patient may be remarkably undistressed despite being critically ill.

● Classical signs are not always present and arterial blood gases are essential for the definitive diagnosis of respiratory failure.

● Patients with respiratory failure may be confused or aggressive. They should *never* be sedated without specialist supervision, e.g. prior to assisted ventilation.

- Obtain a history from relative(s) regarding functional ability at home and numbers of previous admissions (including episodes of mechanical ventilation).
- In patients with chronic respiratory failure a very small insult can provoke severe acute respiratory failure.
- Potentially remediable conditions such as pulmonary oedema, pneumothorax, bronchoconstriction, rib fractures, pleural effusion, and central nervous system depression (due to sedatives or hypnotics) should be excluded as causes for decompensation.
- An altered conscious level and/or inability to cough are unfavourable signs.

Investigations

Chest x-ray
- Look specifically for:
  - Pneumothorax.
  - Signs of infection (collapse, consolidation).
  - Rib fractures.
  - Pulmonary oedema.
  - Pleural effusion(s).

Arterial blood gases
- Signs of hypoxaemia (cyanosis and confusion) and hypercapnia (confusion, drowsiness, flapping tremor, bounding peripheral pulses and dilated peripheral

veins) may be helpful if present but are unreliable.
- A PaO_2 of 6.0 kPa or less (on air) indicates marked hypoxaemia.
- The $[H^+]$ of the arterial blood gas is a useful indicator of the degree of decompensation and if greater than 55 nmol/l should be regarded as suggestive of serious decompensation.
- Previous arterial blood gas records can be extremely valuable in the initial assessment as a severe stable bronchitic may normally have a raised $PaCO_2$ without acidaemia, due to the renal compensatory mechanism.

Management

Airway
- If the airway patency is in doubt, the patient should be intubated and tracheal suction performed.

Oxygen
- Once arterial blood gases have been taken the patient should be put on a low concentration (24–28%) of inspired oxygen via face mask and observed to ensure that the mask is kept on.
- Repeat arterial blood gas sampling about 20–30 minutes after the institution of oxygen therapy.
- It can be dangerous to be overcautious about oxygen therapy, the aim should be to maintain a PaO_2 of 6 kPa

or more without causing a marked rise in the $PaCO_2$ and the resultant acidaemia.

- However, if oxygen therapy results in further hypercapnia, acidaemia, and reduction in conscious level, then the decision regarding the introduction of respiratory stimulants or mechanical ventilation must be made (see below).

Reversible factors

The following should be sought and appropriately treated:

- Retention of secretions.
- Infection.
- Bronchospasm.
- Pneumothorax, rib fractures.
- Pulmonary oedema, pleural effusion.
- Narcotisation with opiate or opiate-like drugs.

'Respiratory stimulants'

- These drugs are not substitutes for airway care.
- They are generalized analeptic agents and may cause acute dysphoric reactions or fitting.
- Nikethamide may be useful in moribund patients. It is given as a 0.5–1.5 mg bolus i.v. with tracheal suction and physiotherapy available.
- Doxapram: a doxapram infusion can be a useful adjuvant to therapy particularly:

•Where there is a defined acute precipitating factor, e.g. central nervous system depressant drugs.

•In those patients with a rise in Pa_{CO_2} and [H$^+$] after institution of oxygen therapy. Dosage: 1.5–2.5 mg/min as an i.v. infusion.

Artificial ventilation

•An anaesthetic specialist should always be informed whenever a patient with severe respiratory failure is admitted.

•Suitable patients may be ventilated if:
  •They are moribund on admission.
  •There is failure of clinical and/or arterial blood gas response to oxygen therapy, tracheal suction, bronchodilators and doxapram.

PULMONARY OEDEMA

Clinical features

•In severe cases, a history of severe dyspnoea, orthopnoea, and a cough is common. Such patients are usually distressed with cool, clammy extremities, central cyanosis, low volume peripheral pulses, dullness on percussion of lung bases, and reduced air entry with late inspiratory crepitations on auscultation.

- In less florid cases, the diagnosis may be indicated by the following points:
  - A history of progressive dyspnoea on exertion and/or nocturnal dyspnoea and orthopnoea (note, however, that asthmatic/bronchitic patients may also exhibit orthopnoea, as when supine they are unable fully to use their accessory respiratory muscles).
  - A past history or clinical features of ischaemic or rheumatic heart disease, hypertension, or renal disease.
  - Inadequate or poor compliance with diuretic therapy, or drugs which may provoke or aggravate left ventricular failure, e.g. β-blockers, non-steroidal anti-inflammatory agents.

Investigations

Chest x-ray

- The most discriminatory investigation in mild/moderate cases.
- Prominent upper zone vessels, basal haziness, Kerley's B lines and cardiomegaly may be present.

12 lead electrocardiogram

- May show patterns of recent myocardial infarction, ischaemia, ventricular hypertrophy, and arrhythmias.

Arterial blood gases
- May be useful in assessing the functional effect of left ventricular failure, but are not discriminatory, as similar results may occur in such conditions as asthma or pulmonary embolism.

Management
- The following steps should be progressively employed according to the clinical state and response of the patient:
  - Sit patient upright.
  - Administer a high concentration (40–60%) of inspired oxygen via face mask. If the patient has a past history of airways disease, repeat arterial blood gases after 15–30 minutes to exclude developing hypercapnia.
  - Give an i.v. short-acting 'loop' diuretic, e.g. frusemide (if the patient is not regularly taking diuretics, an appropriate dose is 40 mg frusemide as a bolus; if the patient is taking regular diuretic therapy up to 250 mg given slowly over 15–20 minutes may be required).
  - Give i.v. morphine titrated slowly to the clinical response (usual dose 2.5–10 mg).
- If the patient is 'in extremis' the following may be required:

• Venesection 500–1000 ml (unless the patient is clinically anaemic).
• Endotracheal intubation and assisted ventilation with positive end-expiratory pressure.

Note

Patients with acute renal failure or those on regular dialysis with salt and water overload before their next dialysis may need opiates and assisted ventilation prior to emergency dialysis. In such cases, venesection is contraindicated and i.v. diuretics are of little value.

PNEUMOTHORAX

Clinical features

• Sudden onset of pleuritic chest pain and/or dyspnoea.
• May occur *de novo*, or following trauma, coughing, or straining.
• On auscultation of the chest, unilateral reduction in air entry and breath sounds may be present. Pleural 'clicks' are occasionally heard and on percussion, hyper-resonance may be detected.
• Rarely displacement of the apex beat, or subcutaneous emphysema may be present.

Investigation

Chest x-ray
- Good quality erect inspiratory and expiratory radiographs are essential.
- Look specifically for:
  - Lung edges.
  - Deviation of trachea or mediastinum.
  - Bullae.

Management

- A 'significant' pneumothorax on chest x-ray (i.e. greater than 30% of total lung field) particularly if associated with dyspnoea, indicates the need for intercostal chest drain insertion (see page 158). However, smaller pneumothoraces may require drainage in patients with chronic chest disease.
- If a patient is 'in extremis' with signs of a tension pneumothorax, insert a wide-bore cannula, e.g. 12–14G, into the second intercostal space in mid-clavicular line. If 'tension' is present, a hiss of escaping air will occur and allow time for formal chest drain insertion.

PULMONARY THROMBOEMBOLISM

- The clinical diagnosis may be very difficult but should be considered in any acutely breathless patient.

- In a potentially life-threatening situation, the patient with 'atypical' features should be regarded as having a pulmonary embolus and started on therapy until the diagnosis can be proven.
- Small peripheral emboli which cause local pleuritic chest pain may be considered separately from massive pulmonary emboli which usually have marked haemo-dynamic effects (see page 39).

MAJOR EMBOLI

- Classical clinical features include a history of sudden onset of dyspnoea, retrosternal chest pain, and, on examination, features of shock with central cyanosis, tachycardia, and an elevated jugular venous pressure.
- 'Atypical' cases are, however, common and one should have a high index of suspicion in the following clinical situations:
  - Any patient with acute dyspnoea especially if cyanosed and without gross signs on examination or chest x-ray to account for the dyspnoea.
  - An apparently 'hysterical' dyspnoeic patient, particularly if arterial blood gases show any degree of hypoxia.
  - Patients presenting with symptoms suggestive of myocardial ischaemia or infarction and dyspnoea but in whom the clinical signs are more related to the

right side of the heart, e.g. elevated jugular venous pressure, fourth heart sound. This is particularly so if there are few signs of left ventricular failure on clinical or radiological examination of the chest.
•A young patient presenting as a 'cardiac arrest'.

Investigations

Chest x-ray
•The chest x-ray may show *no* abnormality.
•Oligaemic lung fields, prominent hilar vessels, and cardiomegaly may be present following major embolism. 'Plate' atelectasis, elevated hemidiaphragms, and small pleural effusions may be present following smaller peripheral emboli.

12 lead electrocardiogram
•The electrocardiogram may show *no* abnormality.
•In major embolism the following features may be present:
  •Sinus tachycardia or atrial arrhythmias (especially atrial fibrillation).
  •Features of acute right heart 'strain' (viz. right bundle branch block, $S_1Q_3T_3$ pattern, inverted T waves in chest leads V_{1-4}).

Arterial blood gases
- Hypoxia, with or without hypocapnia (secondary to hyperventilation) may be present, but is of no diagnostic value.

Management

- Give a high concentration (40–60%) of inspired oxygen via face mask.
- Insert an i.v. cannula.
- If analgesia is required, cautiously give i.v. morphine titrated against response (usual dose 2.5–10 mg).
- Seek specialist advice before giving heparin or other agents, e.g. thrombolytic therapy.
- If a patient with a suspected massive pulmonary embolus has a 'cardiac arrest', commence and continue ventilation and cardiac message, as this may break up or push the embolus peripherally, allowing the patient to survive until emergency angiography/ surgery can be performed.

PSYCHOGENIC DYSPNOEA

- Hysterical hyperventilation can be dramatic and alarming in presentation.
- The patient (usually young) is acutely distressed and apparently dyspnoeic but is *never* cyanosed.

- Marked carpopedal spasm is commonly present.
- Arterial blood gases show normal or slightly elevated Pa_{O_2}. The Pa_{CO_2} will be low with a reduced $[H^+]$.

Management

- The vicious circle can be broken by reassurance together with the patient rebreathing into a paper bag.
- If any atypical features exist in a patient who is 'hysterically hyperventilating', e.g. arterial blood gases showing *any* degree of hypoxia or the patient failing to respond to the above therapy, seek specialist advice as such a patient may, for example, have a pulmonary embolus and will appear (understandably) hysterical.

ANAPHYLACTIC REACTIONS

Anaphylactic reactions may occur in the Accident and Emergency Department:
- Following antitetanus prophylaxis or antibiotic injections.
- In relation to general or local anaesthetics.
- Following the administration of i.v. contrast media.
- During the infusion of plasma, volume expanders, blood, and other blood products.

- *De novo* following exposure to an (un)recognized antigenic stimulus, e.g. non-steroidal anti-inflammatory drugs (especially aspirin) in asthmatic patients, bee or wasp stings.

CLINICAL FEATURES

Respiratory

- Upper airway obstruction—hoarseness and stridor may develop as a result of angio-oedema involving hypopharynx, epiglottis, and larynx.
- Lower airway obstruction—the patient may have subjective feelings of restrosternal tightness and dyspnoea with an audible expiratory wheeze related to bronchospasm.

Cardiovascular

- Features may vary from sinus tachycardia alone to profound hypotension in association with ventricular or supraventricular tachyarrhythmias.
- Rarely, severe bradyarrhythmias (also causing secondary alterations to conscious level as a consequence of hypoperfusion) may occur.

Skin

•The appearance of the skin may be pathognomonic, with the rapid development of urticarial lesions — well circumscribed, intensely pruritic cutaneous weals with erythematous raised edges and blanched centres.

MANAGEMENT

•Upper airway angio-oedema may necessitate prompt endotracheal intubation.
•If the patient's condition is deteriorating and intubation is technically difficult, tracheotomy using one or two large cannulae (12–14G) will permit sufficient ventilation to occur while preparations are made for urgent skilled tracheostomy to be performed.
•Administer oxygen in as high an inspired concentration as can be achieved via face mask.
•Treat bronchospasm if present, by nebulized salbutamol (see page 102).
•Insert an i.v. cannula and attach patient to a cardiac monitor.
•Give 10 mg chlorpheniramine followed by 200 mg hydrocortisone intravenously.
•If the patient's condition is deteriorating give 0.5 ml of 1:1000 adrenaline by deep i.m. or very slow i.v.

injection. This may be repeated up to a total of 2 ml if necessary, but beware cardiac arrhythmias.

●If the patient remains hypotensive, infuse 500 ml 0.9% saline over 15 minutes, then reassess the clinical status.

●Refer for specialist advice, as even if the patient's symptoms and signs have dramatically improved, further observation will be required.

DIABETIC EMERGENCIES

HYPOGLYCAEMIA

General features

●Although hypoglycaemia most commonly occurs in diabetic patients, other groups of patients who may present with hypoglycaemia include those with:
  •A history of recent alcohol ingestion.
  •Previous gastric surgery or liver disease.
  •Accidental or deliberate overdosage with insulin or oral hypoglycaemic agents.

●Confused or aggressive behaviour is a common early feature.

●Subsequently an altered conscious level and bizarre neurological signs, e.g. fits, hemiplegia, may develop.

●Signs of autonomic activity (sweating, tachycardia, pupillary dilation) are common.

Investigation

- Check blood glucose using reagent strips. If a reading of 3 mmol/l or less is obtained, check a blood glucose level formally and while awaiting the result, commence treatment as below.

Management

- Administer dextrose. The route of administration will depend upon the patient's conscious level. Doses:
  - i.v., 50–100 ml 50% dextrose.
  - Oral, 50 g dextrose dissolved in water.
- Following administration of dextrose, the signs of hypoglycaemia should be promptly corrected. However, in those patients who have taken excess insulin (especially if long-acting) or oral hypoglycaemic agents, a prolonged dextrose infusion may be required and specialist help should be obtained.
- Following severe prolonged hypoglycaemia, the patient's conscious level occasionally remains obtunded despite the restoration of normoglycaemia. This may be due to associated conditions, e.g. cerebral oedema or electrolyte disturbances, and specialist advice must be obtained.

120

DIABETIC KETOACIDOSIS AND NON-KETOTIC HYPEROSMOLAR STATES

General features

- The initial management and investigations required for these conditions can be considered together.
- They may be the mode of presentation of patients with previously unrecognized diabetes, or be precipitated in known diabetics by:
  - Local or systemic infection.
  - Tissue infarction, e.g. myocardial, pulmonary, or mesenteric.
  - Any systemic illness.
- While the terms ketoacidosis and non-ketotic hyperosmolar states represent opposing metabolic ends of a spectrum of diabetic disequilibration, their clinical presentations are rarely so clear cut.
- So-called 'classical' features include:

	Ketoacidosis	Non-ketotic hyperosmolar states
Age of patient	Usually <40 years	Usually >40 years
Current diabetic therapy	Insulin-dependent	Non-insulin-dependent

Duration of symptoms	Hours–days	Days–weeks
Signs of salt and water depletion	+ — + + +	+ + +
Ketones detectable on breath/blood/urine	+ + +	o— +
Conscious state	Variable	Variable
Küssmaul respiration	+ — + + +	o— +

Investigations

- Take venous blood samples for the determination of:
  - Urea and electrolytes.
  - Plasma glucose.
  - Full blood count.
  - Blood cultures.
- Take blood for arterial blood gas analysis.
- Chest x-ray.
- 12 lead electrocardiogram and attach patient to a cardiac monitor.

Management

- If the patient has altered consciousness, ensure the airway and the ventilation is adequate, pass a nasogastric tube and aspirate the stomach.
- Insert an i.v. cannula.

- The rate of infusion of i.v. fluids will depend upon the severity of the patient's clinical condition. Central venous pressure monitoring may assist in the assessment and therapeutic response and should be particularly considered in the elderly, or those patients with myocardial disease. However, in general, 1000 ml of 0.9% saline should be administered over the first hour.
- Give a loading dose of 4 units of soluble insulin i.v. followed by 6 units as an infusion over the first hour.
- The rate and content of further i.v. fluids (including potassium and bicarbonate administration) will depend upon laboratory information and the patient's clinical state. Early specialist advice should be obtained.

FITS, COLLAPSES, AND STATES OF ALTERED CONSCIOUSNESS

COMMON CAUSES

- Vasovagal episode.
- Epilepsy.
- Hypoglycaemia.
- Postural hypotension.
- Drug overdose.

LESS COMMON CAUSES

- Subarachnoid haemorrhage.
- Cerebrovascular accident/transient ischaemic attack.
- Ischaemic heart disease (arrhythmias/myocardial ischaemia or infarction).
- Meningitis/encephalitis.
- Metabolic causes (hepatic/renal failure, Addison's disease).
- 'Silent' gastrointestinal haemorrhage.
- Micturition or cough syncope.

HISTORY

- Ask eye-witness specifically about:
  - Preceding events, including trauma.
  - The episode itself:
    - Changes in consciousness and their duration.
    - (Abnormal) movements of face, limbs.
    - Skin colour changes.
    - Trauma sustained during the episode.
    - Possibility of aspiration.
- Ask the patient about:
  - Precipitating events:
    - Posture changes.
    - Head turning.
    - Coughing, straining, micturition.

    ·Exposure to flashing lights or television.
·Cardiovascular symptoms:
  ·Dyspnoea.
  ·Chest pain/tightness.
  ·Palpitations.
·Current drug therapy:
  ·Antihypertensive agents, antiarrhythmic drugs, glyceryl trinitrate, diuretics.
  ·Sedatives, antidepressant drugs, L-dopa.
  ·Insulin, oral hypoglycaemic agents, steroids.
·Use of alcohol, opiates, or other drugs.
·Past medical history:
  ·Previous similar episodes.
  ·Ischaemic and/or rheumatic heart disease.
  ·Diabetes, epilepsy, or gastric surgery.
  ·Recent infections or vaccinations.
•Obtain further history from patient's general practitioner or relatives.

EXAMINATION

Airway

•Look for signs of vomiting/aspiration, tongue biting, gum hypertrophy.
•Smell breath for ketones, alcohol, hepatic or uraemic foetor.
•Note the respiratory pattern and auscultate chest.

Cardiovascular system

- Pulse rate, rhythm.
- Blood pressure (erect and supine if possible).
- Peripheral perfusion, skin colour, sweating, and capillary filling.
- Auscultate heart, in particular for evidence of aortic/ mitral valve disease. Listen for carotid, cranial, or abdominal bruits.

Central nervous system

- Assess conscious level (using Glasgow coma scale).
- Look for neck stiffness and/or photophobia.
- Examine the cranial nerves (including examination of the optic fundi and external auditory meatus).
- Assess muscle tone, power, sensation, and tendon reflexes.

General

- Look for signs of trauma, blood loss, bruising, pressure marks, incontinence.
- Assess the state of hydration.
- Measure temperature. If oral or axillary temperature is less than 35 °C, check the reading rectally.
- Look for needle puncture marks on arms, the inguinal area, thighs, and genitalia.

- Look for medical identification bracelets/lockets/key rings, steroid/diabetic cards or drug bottles.

INVESTIGATIONS

- Check blood glucose using reagent strips: if the reading is greater than 10 mmol/l, send blood for formal laboratory measurement of plasma glucose and urea and electrolytes. If reading is less than 3 mmol/l, see page 118.
- 12-lead electrocardiogram: look for arrhythmias, signs of ischaemia/infarction. If the electrocardiogram is normal and the patient has no carotid bruits nor neurological/cardiovascular signs or symptoms, perform carotid sinus massage alternately on both sides of the neck while the electrocardiograph trace is running.
- Carotid sinus hypersensitivity is present if the ventricular rate slows to 30 or less per minute, or the patient develops related symptoms. (Transient) asystole or nodal escape rhythms may occur.
- In any patient who has altered consciousness without a clear-cut cause, give 0.8 mg i.v. naloxone. A dramatic response to this implies intoxication with an opiate or opiate-like drug (see page 146).
- Other investigations which may be indicated:
  - X-ray of chest/skull.
  - Urea and electrolytes.

- Arterial blood gases.
- Breath/blood alcohol levels.
- Anticonvulsant levels.

VASOVAGAL EPISODE

- Commonly occurs in stressful, warm environments, particularly if the patient is erect.
- Prodromal dizziness, nausea, pallor, and sweating are often present.
- The patient recovers rapidly when placed in a supine position.

THE FITTING PATIENT

The commonest causes of fitting in the Accident and Emergency Department are:
- Epilepsy.
- Drug/alcohol: withdrawal or overdose.
- Intracranial event:
  - Subarachnoid haemorrhage.
  - 'Stroke'.
  - Meningitis/encephalitis.
  - Hypertensive encephalopathy.
- Following the administration of drugs in the department (e.g. local anaesthetic agents).

Management

• Maintain the patient's airway and ventilation appropriately.
• Control of the fit:
  • Rarely the fit is caused or related to hypoxia, hypoglycaemia or severe hypo/hypertension. If present, these conditions should be appropriately corrected.
  • Give diazepam in aliquots of 2.5 mg by i.v. route (rarely more than 20 mg is required).
  • If there is no response to these measures, the patient may have to be paralysed and ventilated. Specialist advice should be obtained before this is undertaken.

EPILEPSY

• In patients with an epileptic tendency fits may be precipitated by:
  • Hypoglycaemia.
  • Infection.
  • Drug/alcohol withdrawal or intoxication.
  • Visual/auditory stimuli.
• In patients on anticonvulsant therapy, an increase in fit frequency may be related to supra- or subtherapeutic levels.
• A known epileptic patient who has an isolated fit can be discharged home if:

·He did not sustain related trauma requiring referral.
·He rapidly regained consciousness with no residual neurological signs.
·He can be supervised by a family member or friend.
●First fits, multiple or frequent fits, incomplete recovery with neurological sequelae (e.g. Todd's paralysis) or fits related to trauma or infection will require specialist referral.

HYPOGLYCAEMIA

See page 118.

POSTURAL HYPOTENSION

●History is usually related to changes in position from the supine posture.
●It commonly presents in the elderly, diabetic or Addisonian patients and those on antihypertensive drugs.
●A fall of 30 mmHg or more in systolic blood pressure between supine and erect positions together with subjective symptoms is pathognomonic.

DRUG OVERDOSE

The possibility of acute or chronic drug overdose should always be considered as a cause of altered consciousness (see page 140).

SUBARACHNOID HAEMORRHAGE

- Although a classical history (sudden severe headache, collapse, photophobia) is common, signs (including neck stiffness) may be absent.
- Look for evidence of vascular disease/hypertension.
- Refer for specialist inpatient investigation and management.

TRANSIENT ISCHAEMIC ATTACKS

- Common symptoms include temporary episodes of visual loss, dysphasia, unilateral motor/sensory loss or vertigo.
- Look for evidence of vascular disease and possible sources of emboli, e.g. carotid bruits, valve prostheses, previous myocardial infarction. Remember that patients with mitral stenosis run risk of emboli even in sinus rhythm.
- Obtain specialist advice regarding referral.

ARRHYTHMIAS

- A history of palpitations or sudden collapse with absent pulses and the spontaneous return of consciousness may be the only pointer to the diagnosis.
- A 12 lead electrocardiogram may be entirely normal

between symptomatic episodes. Occasionally, abnormalities such as the Wolff–Parkinson–White or sick sinus syndromes are found.
- Look for signs of aortic/mitral valve disease.
- If it is suspected that the collapse is due to an arrhythmia, specialist referral for 24 hour electrocardiogram taping or elective pacing is indicated.

CAROTID SINUS HYPERSENSITIVITY
- The symptoms are often related to head-turning particularly in elderly patients.
- Specialist referral for consideration of permanent cardiac pacing is indicated.

MYOCARDIAL ISCHAEMIA/INFARCTION
(see page 87).
- 'Silent' myocardial events may occur particularly in elderly or diabetic patients.
- Remember that aortic stenosis or obstructive cardiomyopathies can result in exertional syncope or ischaemic chest pain in patients of all ages.

MENINGITIS AND ENCEPHALITIS
- There may be a history of recent infection or head injury.

● Look for skin rashes, signs of meningeal irritation, and/or raised intracranial pressure.
● Specialist referral is indicated.

HYPOTHERMIA AND DROWNING

HYPOTHERMIA

● The following groups of patients are at particular risk of developing hypothermia:
  · The elderly.
  · Those with altered consciousness.
  · Those with conditions commonly causing inactivity, e.g. Parkinson's disease, crippling illnesses, hypothyroidism.
  · Following alcohol ingestion and/or drug overdose.
  · Those exposed to low ambient temperatures or immersion in water.
● Take the patient's temperature rectally using a low-reading thermometer.
● Remember that the clinical signs of death in patients with severe hypothermia can be misleading. In such cases continue full resuscitation until core temperature is greater than 35 °C, or specialist advice has been sought, before declaring such a patient to be dead.

Examination

General
- Skin colour, bruising, peripheral cyanosis.
- Peripheral oedema.
- Presence of ketones or alcohol on breath.

Systematic
- Pulse rate, rhythm, and blood pressure.
- Note respiratory rate and pattern and auscultate chest to detect the commonly associated features of pulmonary oedema and/or pneumonia.
- Conscious level.
- Muscular tone, briskness, and symmetry of tendon reflexes and pupillary reactions.

Investigations

- Arterial blood gases (remember to inform the laboratory of patient's temperature to allow for appropriate correction to be calculated).
- 12 lead electrocardiogram and cardiac monitor: arrhythmias (especially atrial fibrillation and/or bradyarrhythmias) are common. Associated conduction defects and J waves may also be present.
- Chest x-ray.
- Send appropriate blood samples for urea and electrolytes,

plasma glucose and amylase estimations (disorders of plasma potassium and hypoglycaemia are common and an associated pancreatitis may be present).

Management

- Ensure an adequate airway and administer a high concentration (40–60%) of inspired oxygen.
- Handling of the patient should be kept to a minimum as arrhythmias may be precipitated; thus, in general, unless the patient is apnoeic, it is best to avoid endotracheal intubation.
- Insert an i.v. cannula. If i.v. fluids are given, they should be warmed to 37 °C prior to administration.
- Correct any acidosis using 20 ml aliquots of 8.4% sodium bicarbonate (the total amount given should be guided by the patient's clinical state in association with repeated arterial blood gas analysis).
- If the patient is hypotensive and doubt as to circulating volume status exists, a central venous pressure line should be inserted. Sequential readings of the central venous pressure usually help to prevent the inappropriate administration of large volumes of i.v. fluid.
- Remember that drugs given by oral or i.m. routes will be incompletely and erratically absorbed.

Rewarming

- Nurse in a warm environment.
- Prevent further heat loss by covering the patient with polythene sheets or a 'space blanket'.
- Do not apply heat directly to the skin.
- If core temperature is less than 30 °C, urgently call for specialist help and consider active rewarming by immersion of the trunk in a warm bath at 40 °C, or peritoneal/mediastinal lavage with warmed fluid.

Prevent or Treat Complications

Arrhythmias
- Prevent by gentle handling.
- Arrhythmias (especially atrial fibrillation) are common but rarely need specific treatment and will revert to normal sinus rhythm with correction of hypothermia.
- Bradyarrhythmias will usually respond to atropine given i.v. (dose: 0.6–1.2 mg).

Hypotension
- Keep patient supine.
- In the absence of hypovolaemia due to associated conditions, e.g. diabetes mellitus, do not attempt to 'correct' hypotension by infusing i.v. fluids.

Pulmonary oedema
- Prevent by avoiding excessive i.v. fluid administration.
- Treat with i.v. frusemide and administer a high concentration (40–60%) of inspired oxygen if pulmonary oedema has developed.

DROWNING

Clinical features

- A precipitating cause for the episode, e.g. drug/alcohol intoxication, head injury, is commonly present and should be sought and treated appropriately.
- The patient must be examined for injuries sustained before, during, or after the fall into the water.
- Hypothermia frequently results as a consequence of immersion in water.
- Sudden immersion into (cold) water may result in brady- or tachyarrhythmias, cardiac arrest, myocardial ischaemia/infarction or cerebrovascular 'accidents'.
- If water or other liquids are inhaled, hypoxia is an early consequence. However, signs of pulmonary oedema and the adult respiratory distress syndrome can develop up to 72 hours following the initial event.
- The nature of the inhaled liquid, e.g. salt or fresh water, does not alter the initial assessment and management of such patients.

Investigations

- A 12 lead electrocardiogram may show associated arrhythmias or features of acute myocardial ischaemia or infarction.
- Chest x-ray: look specifically for evidence of aspiration (in the early stages this is often manifest as patchy opacification occurring in both lung fields).
- Arterial blood gases: hypoxia and a mixed respiratory/metabolic acidosis are commonly present.
- Blood should be sent for laboratory estimation of urea and electrolytes. Plasma sodium/potassium abnormalities can occur but are rarely present in the early stages of management.

Management

- The initial management is very similar to that for the hypothermic patient. However, because of the nature of the condition, endotracheal intubation and assisted ventilation will often be required.
- In such cases, specialist advice should be obtained regarding positive pressure ventilation, as this may improve gas exchange and prevent later complications.

HYPERTENSIVE EMERGENCIES

CLINICAL FEATURES

- Always check the patient's blood pressure in both arms yourself.
- Look for signs/consequences of acute or chronic hypertension:
  - Fundal changes.
  - Cardiomegaly.
  - Bruits.
- Look for evidence of left ventricular failure.
- Is there an acutely remedial or causative factor, for example:
  - Recently discontinued medication (e.g. clonidine, β-blocking agents) or drug interaction (e.g. monoamine oxidase inhibitor and tricyclic antidepressant agents or tyramine).
  - Intracranial pathology.
  - Coarctation of the aorta, phaeochromocytoma, renal disease.

INVESTIGATIONS

- Cardiac monitor.
- 12 lead electrocardiogram.
- Chest x-ray.

- Urinalysis.
- Send venous blood sample for determination of urea and electrolytes.

MANAGEMENT

- Hypertension *per se* is *not* an indication for therapeutic intervention in the Accident and Emergency Department.
- The rapid lowering of blood pressure may result in irreversible cardio- or cerebrovascular disasters.

If patient is well

- Monitor the patient's vital signs and general condition closely.
- Resist the temptation to dabble therapeutically!
- Refer for inpatient care.

If patient has evidence of cardiac failure

- Give high (40–60%) inspired concentration of oxygen via face mask.
- Give i.v. frusemide (dosage will depend upon the clinical severity of cardiac failure and the patient's current therapy, but usually between 20 and 120 mg is required).

- If required, give i.v. morphine, titrated against clinical response.
- Refer for inpatient care.

If patient has associated central nervous system disturbance, e.g. fits, altered consciousness, visual disturbance

- Ensure adequate airway and ventilation.
- Fitting should be treated with diazepam given by slow i.v. injection, dosage to be titrated against response (usual dose 5–20 mg).
- Treat cardiac failure, if present, as above.
- Seek specialist advice regarding the use of specific hypotensive agents. (Sodium nitroprusside given by infusion, 0.5–5 μg/kg/min, may be valuable in this situation. This agent will act within 1–3 minutes of administration and has a very short half-life so that the infusion rate can be closely titrated against the therapeutic response.)

POISONING

HISTORY

- To which drug(s), poison(s) or substance(s) has the patient been exposed?:

- •When?
- •By what route(s)?
- •Why?
- ●Has the patient vomited since intake/exposure?

GENERAL POINTS

- ●In the severely poisoned patient, history, examination, and resuscitation should be performed simultaneously.
- ●Consider the possibility of coexistent disease or secondary effects related to the episode itself, e.g. hypothermia, muscle or thermal injury.
- ●Ensure that the patient is fully undressed and examined particularly for:
  - •Needle punctures.
  - •Bruising or blistering.
  - •Colour of mucous membranes.
  - •(Self-inflicted) wounds.
  - •Signs of vomiting and aspiration.

INVESTIGATIONS

- ●Check blood glucose using reagent strips and send blood samples for formal laboratory measurement of plasma glucose and urea and electrolytes.
- ●Arterial blood gases and a chest x-ray should be performed if any doubt exists as to the adequacy of

ventilation, or if there is any possibility of exposure to smoke, inhaled chemicals, or aspiration.
- A 12 lead electrocardiogram should be performed and the patient attached to a cardiac monitor.
- Samples for measurement of drug/toxin levels can conveniently be taken and sent at this stage, but play little role in the immediate care of such patients.

MANAGEMENT

General points

- Few cases of poisoning will require more than the provision of an adequate airway, ventilation, and supportive nursing and medical care, in their immediate resuscitation.
- An i.v. cannula (either flushed with heparinized saline and occluded, or kept open with a slow infusion of 0.9% saline) should be inserted to permit venous access.
- Although patients poisoned with substances such as aspirin, paracetamol, metals, etc., rarely present to the Accident and Emergency Department in a life-threatening state, the appropriate antidote, gastric lavage, or other therapy may be required within a given time from drug ingestion if it is to be effective. In all cases immediate life-saving measures should

be taken and the patient promptly referred to the appropriate specialist.

- If the patient has associated fitting, maintain airway and ventilation and give i.v. diazepam slowly titrated against response (dose usually required 5–20 mg).
- Poison centres (see page 173) are available for immediate advice regarding management or complications.

SPECIFIC POISONS

β-blockers

- In severe overdosage, bradyarrhythmias (or even asystole) and electrolyte disturbances are common.
- Give a high (40–60%) concentration of inspired oxygen via face mask and airway care as necessary.
- In the presence of a low cardiac output state as a consequence of bradyarrhythmias:
  - Give i.v. atropine (dose: 1.2 mg administered as a bolus. This may be repeated once if required.) If no response:
  - Give i.v. glucagon (dose: 2 mg aliquots administered as bolus doses up to a total of 10 mg). If no response:
  - Give as isoprenaline infusion (dosage to be titrated to heart rate and clinical response (see page 26).
  - Continued failure of clinical response may indicate

the need for urgent cardiac pacing under specialist supervision.

Carbon monoxide

- Poisoning with carbon monoxide is usually related to exposure to exhaust fumes or incomplete combustion of domestic gas.
- The classical 'cherry-red' appearance of mucous membranes is not always obvious. Other clinical features may include altered consciousness, haematemesis, hypotension, cardiac arrhythmias, and neurological deficits.
- Check arterial blood gases and carboxyhaemoglobin level.
- Administer oxygen in as high an inspired concentration as can be achieved.
- Correct gross acid–base disturbances appropriately.
- If the patient is unconscious, give 100–200 ml of 20% mannitol to prevent or reduce the effects of associated cerebral oedema.

Cyanide

- The clinical features of severe cyanide poisoning may include loss of consciousness, fitting, hypotension, cardiac arrhythmias, and pulmonary oedema.

- The treatment of cyanide poisoning is itself potentially toxic and should only be given to patients with signs of moderate–severe poisoning.
- The antidote of choice is i.v. dicobalt edetate (dose 300 mg administered over 60 seconds. A further 300 mg can be given if there is no improvement after 1–2 minutes).

Insulin or hypoglycaemic agents

- Signs of severe hypoglycaemia (see page 118) will usually be present.
- Give 50% dextrose i.v. (up to 150 ml may be initially required). Subsequently a continuous infusion of 10–20% dextrose may be required for hours/days depending upon the dose and half-life of the agent taken.
- Do not be misled by the apparent complete restoration of conscious levels and vital signs after the initial correction of hypoglycaemia. Complications such as cerebral oedema, cerebrovascular 'accidents', etc., may occur.
- Occasionally, following severe overdosage with oral hypoglycaemic agents (e.g. chlorpropamide) there is no response to i.v. dextrose; in such cases seek specialist advice regarding the use of such agents as diazoxide to correct the resistant hypoglycaemia.

Opiates

- Although respiratory depression, altered consciousness, and small pupils classically occur in opiate overdosage, these signs are not invariably present.
- Give 0.8 mg i.v. naloxone immediately.
- The clinical features of opiate overdosage are usually reversed by naloxone within 2–3 minutes. Further i.v. or i.m. doses may be required as the half-life of naloxone is shorter than many opiates and after initial reversal, the patient's condition may relapse owing to continued activity of the opiate.
- The efficacy and safety of naloxone are such that it should be given to any patient who has altered consciousness without a clearly identifiable cause. While minor reversal effects have been noted with other drugs and in some clinical states, a dramatic response to administration of naloxone implies intoxication with an opiate or opiate-like drug.

Salicylates

- Common features of overdosage include tinnitus, deafness, nausea, vomiting, sweating, peripheral vasodilation, and hyperventilation.
- Altered consciousness, fitting, and sudden cardiac arrest are rare but may occur in very severe overdosage.

- Complex metabolic and acid–base disturbances as reflected in arterial blood gas, urea, electrolyte and plasma glucose levels will usually be present.
- Commence an i.v. infusion with 0.9% saline and seek specialist advice regarding the interpretation and correction of these disturbances.

Tricyclic antidepressants

- Common clinical features of overdosage include dilated pupils, dry warm skin, hyperreflexia, muscular twitching, hypotension, and cardiac arrhythmias. Respiratory depression is less common.
- The wide variety of arrhythmias which can occur are generally well tolerated by the patient (even when the electrocardiographic picture is disturbing). The correction of associated hypoxia and acidosis will frequently restore a more 'normal' rhythm.
- If the arrhythmia persists and is poorly tolerated further treatment may be required.

In such cases, specialist advice must be sought, as many standard antiarrhythmic drugs (including β-blockers, lignocaine, digoxin and disopyramide) can potentiate the cardiotoxicity of tricyclic antidepressant drugs.

Section 4

CARDIOVERSION

INDICATIONS

- Ventricular fibrillation.
- Life-threatening tachyarrhythmias, viz. those resulting in haemodynamic embarrassment (hypotension, altered consciousness, myocardial ischaemia, or cardiac failure).

TECHNIQUE

The patient with ventricular fibrillation

- Ensure that the patient *is* unconscious and has no detectable carotid/femoral pulses.
- While the defibrillator is being prepared and charged, cardiopulmonary resuscitation (see page 3) must be commenced and continued until a satisfactory spontaneous cardiac output is achieved.
- Coat the defibrillator paddles with electrode gel and place one over the lower left chest and the other to the right of the upper sternum.
- Check that neither the operator nor other staff are in contact with the patient, the trolley/bed or associated equipment.
- Apply d.c. shock at 200 J.

- If there is no response, recommence ventilation and cardiac massage while recharging the defibrillator. Subsequent d.c. shocks should be repeated at 400 J.
- Concomitant drug therapy may be indicated in cases of refractory ventricular fibrillation (see page 8).

The patient with life-threatening tachyarrhythmias

- Ensure that full resuscitation equipment is immediately available and the patient has an i.v. cannula *in situ*.
- If the patient is conscious seek urgent specialist advice.
- In patients who have lost or altered consciousness, the airway must be appropriately maintained and the patient given a high concentration of inspired oxygen.
- If the patient has altered consciousness with signs of circulatory failure and specialist help is not immediately available, give i.v. diazepam slowly (usual dose 5–20 mg) until the eyelash reflex or response to a moderately severe painful stimulus is depressed. (Remember that the circulation times for drugs given by i.v. route will be prolonged.)
- If the patient is unconscious proceed as below:
  - With the defibrillator on '*synchronized*' mode apply a 50 J shock (remember to keep the 'firing' button depressed until the synchronization mechanism allows the shock to occur on the R wave of the electrocardiogram).

•Note that return to a stable sinus rhythm may be preceded by a few seconds of asystole, bradycardia, or other unstable rhythms. Maintain airway and oxygenation until full recovery of consciousness.

Note

Wherever possible, cardioversion should be avoided in patients taking digoxin due to the possibility of inducing refractory asystole. In such cases if the patient's state necessitates cardioversion, commence with 10 J shocks and increase the energy of subsequent shocks in 20 J steps if required.

CENTRAL VENOUS CANNULATION

INDICATIONS

•A central venous line may be required in an emergency:
  •To permit rapid i.v. access, e.g. cardiac arrest.
  •To permit recordings of central venous pressure.
  •To allow insertion of a transvenous cardiac pacemaker.
•The casualty officer should be familiar with at least one approach to the internal jugular as well as the subclavian vein. The approaches described below are

those that the editors consider to be the simplest and safest.

- •Whenever a central venous line is being inserted:
  - •Full aseptic procedure must be employed.
  - •The patient should be tilted 10–15° head down to increase venous filling and reduce the risk of air embolism.
  - •The vein should be located with a 21G needle before the cannula assembly is introduced. This can be temporarily left *in situ* to provide a directional aid to cannula insertion.
- •Whenever possible cannulate the right subclavian or internal jugular veins (to avoid thoracic duct).

INTERNAL JUGULAR VEIN (MEDIAL APPROACH)

- •The vein runs in a straight line deep to the sterno-mastoid from mastoid process to sternoclavicular joint. It lies in the carotid sheath, lateral to the internal and common carotid arteries.
- •With the patient's head turned to the left, the needle/ cannula should be inserted medial to the line of the vein at its midpoint and at an angle of 30–40° from the horizontal.
- •Advance the needle/cannula in an inferior and slightly lateral direction.

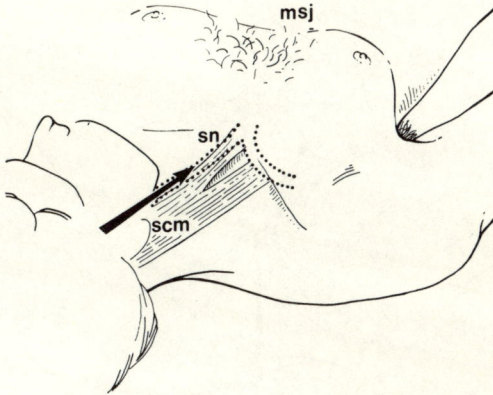

Fig. 19. The medial approach to the internal jugular vein: msj, manubriosternal joint; scm, sternocleidomastoid; sn, sternal notch

•The vein should be entered at a needle depth of 3–4 cm.

SUBCLAVIAN VEIN
(SUPRACLAVICULAR APPROACH)

•The vein runs across the first rib and then behind the medial third of the clavicle to the medial border of the clavicular head of sternomastoid where it joins the internal jugular vein to form the innominate vein. The

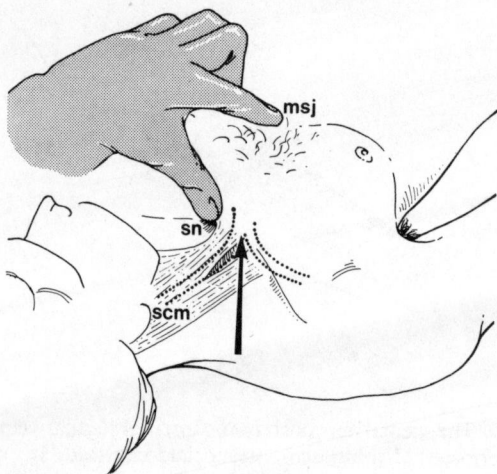

Fig. 20. The supraclavicular approach to the subclavian vein: msj, manubriosternal joint; scm, sternocleidomastoid; sn, sternal notch

vein lies anterior to the subclavian artery and medial to the apical pleura.
• Turn the patient's head to the left. Bisecting the angle between the clavicle and the clavicular head of sterno-mastoid, advance the needle/cannula under the clavicle in a horizontal plane with respect to the patient, towards the manubriosternal joint.

●The vein should be entered at a needle depth of 3–5 cm.

AFTER INSERTION OF THE
CENTRAL VENOUS LINE

●Check that blood can be aspirated from the cannula before fluid is infused.
●Obtain a chest x-ray and check that:
  ·The catheter is correctly positioned.
  ·A pneumo- or haemothorax has not arisen.
●Ensure that the cannula is taped/sutured securely to the skin and that the cannula and giving set cannot become disconnected.
●Check that no neck haematoma (which may compromise airway) is developing.

POSSIBLE PROBLEMS

●If the operator is unable to locate or introduce the cannula into the chosen vein despite two attempts, specialist advice should be sought.
●Provided scrupulous attention is paid to positioning and technique, arterial puncture, haemo- or pneumothorax are uncommon. If these or any other complications occur urgent specialist advice must be sought.

CENTRAL VENOUS PRESSURE MONITORING

- Attach the central venous cannula to a manometer using a three-way tap.
- During measurement of the central venous pressure, check that the fluid level in the manometer swings freely with respiration.
- The central venous pressure should be measured from a defined fixed zero reference point. This is commonly considered to be the right atrium.

CHEST DRAIN INSERTION

INDICATIONS

Pneumothorax

- In general all pneumothoraces secondary to trauma will require drainage.
- Simple spontaneous pneumothorax rarely requires *immediate* drainage unless:
  - The patient is dyspnoeic.
  - There is associated chronic chest disease.
  - Patient requires assisted ventilation.

Haemopneumothorax

Related to trauma.

DIAGNOSIS

- If a tension pneumothorax is clinically apparent immediate needle decompression is required. Otherwise the diagnosis should be made from an erect anteroposterior chest x-ray.
- Remember that bullae or traumatic rupture of the diaphragm can mimic a pneumothorax on chest radiographs. Inspiratory and expiratory films may clarify the situation.

TECHNIQUE

- Recheck clinical and radiological findings relating to the affected side.
- Check the contents of pack and underwater seal connections.
- Explain the procedure to the patient.
- Use full aseptic procedure. Infiltrate the skin and subcutaneous tissues down to the pleura with 1% plain lignocaine using the second intercostal space in the mid-clavicular line (the fourth intercostal space in the mid-axillary line is an alternative site).
- With a scalpel make a 2 cm incision through the skin and intercostal muscles.
- Insert a purse-string suture using 0/0 black silk.
- With firm pressure, and a slight rotatory movement,

introduce the trocar/cannula assembly through the incision. When a "give" is felt, push the cannula into the pleural space while withdrawing the introducer. Kink the tube to prevent further air entering the pleural cavity while the connection to the underwater seal bottle is made.

- After connection, check that bubbles are escaping into the bottle.
- Tie the purse-string suture securely around the tube.
- Pad the wound with swabs, then tape the wound and tube securely to chest.
- Repeat chest x-ray to ensure re-expansion of lung and to locate tube.

POSSIBLE PROBLEMS

Painful introduction

- May be related to associated rib fractures.
- Reinfiltrate the area with lignocaine.
- If there is an underlying flail segment, this may 'give' as the trocar/cannula assembly is pushed in and hinder insertion; ensure that the skin incision is long enough and the intercostal muscles have been incised.

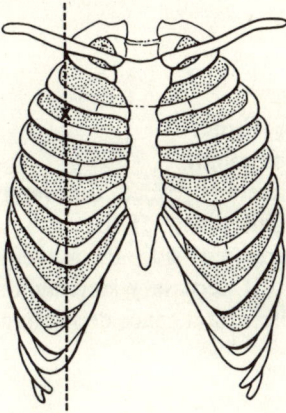 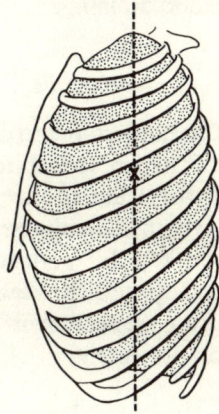

Mid-clavicular line

Mid-axillary line

Fig. 21. Sites for chest drain insertion

Blood coming down drain

- A small amount of blood is not unusual, but greater than 50 ml may indicate a haemothorax or intercostal vessel damage.
- Intercostal vessel damage can be avoided by insertion of the assembly just above the third rib rather than below the second rib where vessels lie.
- Ensure an i.v. line is *in situ* and blood sample is sent for grouping and cross-matching.

●Carefully observe pulse, blood pressure and amount of blood draining.

Non-swinging tube

●Check there are no clamps on tubing.
●Get patient to inspire deeply or cough.
●If the peumothorax is completely absorbed, the water level in the column should still swing. If the tube is blocked lie patient on uninjured side to prevent occlusion of the cannula and if necessary start again using the second or fourth intercostal space depending on first attempt.

PERICARDIOCENTESIS

INDICATION

●Cardiac tamponade.

TECHNIQUE

General points

●Ensure that full resuscitation equipment is immediately available.

- Monitor the electrocardiogram throughout.
- Full aseptic procedure should be followed.

Inferior approach (Fig. 22)

- Patient should sit on a trolley with his back supported at 45°.
- Infiltrate skin and subcutaneous tissues immediately below the xiphoid process with 1% lignocaine.
- Insert a 16G needle attached to a 20 ml syringe (and if possible connected to the chest-lead terminal of an electrocardiograph machine by a crocodile clip) between the xiphoid process and left costal margin at 45° to the patient's long axis. Direct the needle towards the tip of the left shoulder.
- Maintain suction on the syringe. As the needle enters the pericardium, blood will enter the syringe.
- If the needle touches or penetrates the ventricular wall, it will pulsate and the cardiac monitor trace may show elevated ST segment changes.
- Attach a three-way tap to the needle and aspirate to dryness.

PRECAUTIONS AND COMPLICATIONS

- Always perform a chest x-ray after the procedure; look specifically for presence of pneumo- or haemothorax.

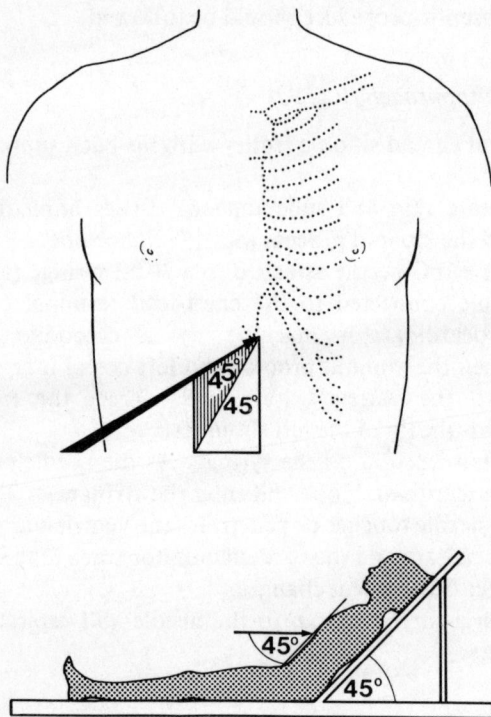

Fig. 22. The inferior approach for aspiration of the pericardium

- Ventricular puncture may provoke arrhythmias, cardiac arrest, or haemopericardium.
- Traumatic haemopericardium is an indication for urgent thoracotomy; pericardiocentesis merely 'buys time' in this situation.

PERITONEAL LAVAGE

INDICATIONS

Peritoneal lavage is used to assess the presence of intra-peritoneal haemorrhage in:
- Patients with multiple injuries (particularly if associated with altered consciousness).
- Patients with an abdominal injury and 'unexplained' hypotension.

TECHNIQUE

- Pass a nasogastric tube and urinary catheter to ensure that stomach and bladder are empty.
- Select site for cannula insertion. If there has been no previous abdominal surgery, the optimal site is in the midline two fingers' breadth below the umbilicus. Alternative sites are in the iliac fossae.

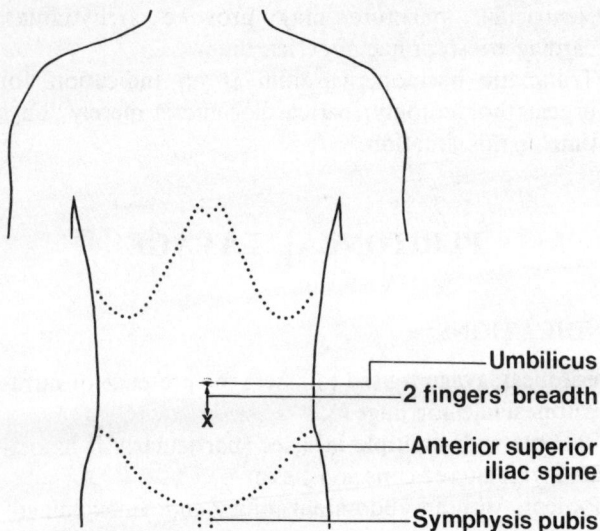

Fig. 23. Site for insertion of peritoneal lavage cannula

- Use a full aseptic procedure.
- Tip the patient 5–10° head down.
- Infiltrate the skin and subcutaneous tissues down to the linea alba with 1% lignocaine and adrenaline solution.
- Make a ½–1 cm incision down to and including the linea alba. Ensure meticulous haemostasis.
- With the left hand, grip the cannula and stylet

assembly by its lower third to control the depth of penetration, and using a twisting motion of the right hand insert through the incision and peritoneum.

- During insertion, angle the assembly posteroinferiorly towards the sacrum. Penetration of the peritoneum is characterized by a 'give'.
- Insert the cannula further into the peritoneum while withdrawing the stylet until all the cannula's holes are in the peritoneal cavity.
- Withdraw the stylet completely. Aspirate using a 20 ml syringe; if blood is freely obtained, no lavage is required.
- Run 1000 ml of warmed 0.9% saline into the peritoneal cavity using an i.v. giving set. Allow the fluid to remain *in situ* for 5 minutes.
- During this time, correct the head-down tilt and if possible gently rock the patient from side to side.
- Place the i.v. infusion bag on the floor and allow the fluid to drain out of the peritoneal cavity under gravity.
- Any blood-staining of the effluent fluid is indicative of intraperitoneal bleeding requiring specialist surgical advice regarding exploration. If weakly blood-stained fluid (which may merely look cloudy) is drained, further lavage with 1000 ml 0.9% saline should be performed. If colour/cloudiness persists, a positive lavage should be assumed.

•After lavage, remove the cannula and close the incision with a suture.

POSSIBLE PROBLEMS

•Rarely, bladder or bowel puncture can occur and will require specialist surgical advice regarding further advice.

•If after insertion, the lavage fluid does not run freely, consider the possibility that the cannula is not within the peritoneal cavity, and if necessary repeat the insertion procedure.

•If the lavage fluid fails to drain freely, drainage may be facilitated by gently changing the patient's position and/or flushing the cannula with 10–20 ml of 0.9% saline.

Appendices

Appendices

DRUG NOMENCLATURE

Generic name	Proprietary name(s)
Chlorpropamide	Diabinese/Glymese/Melitase
Dexamethasone	Decadron Shock Pak/Oradexon
Dextran 70	Lomodex 70/Macrodex
Diazepam	Diazemuls/Valium
Dicobalt edetate	Kelocyanor
Digoxin	Lanoxin
Disopyramide	Norpace/Rythmodan
Dobutamine	Dobutrex
Dopamine	Intropin
Doxapram	Dopram
Frusemide	Dryptal/Lasix
Hydrocortisone	Efcortelan Soluble/Efcortesol/ Solu-Cortef
Lignocaine	Xylocard
Mannitol	Osmitrol
Mexiletine	Mexitil
Naloxone	Narcan
Paracetamol	Calpol/Paldesic/Panadol/ Panasorb/Salzone
Phenytoin	Epanutin
Practolol	Eraldin
Salbutamol	Ventolin
Sodium nitroprusside	Nipride
Terbutaline sulphate	Bricanyl
Verapamil	Cordilox

INTERPRETATION OF ARTERIAL BLOOD GAS DATA

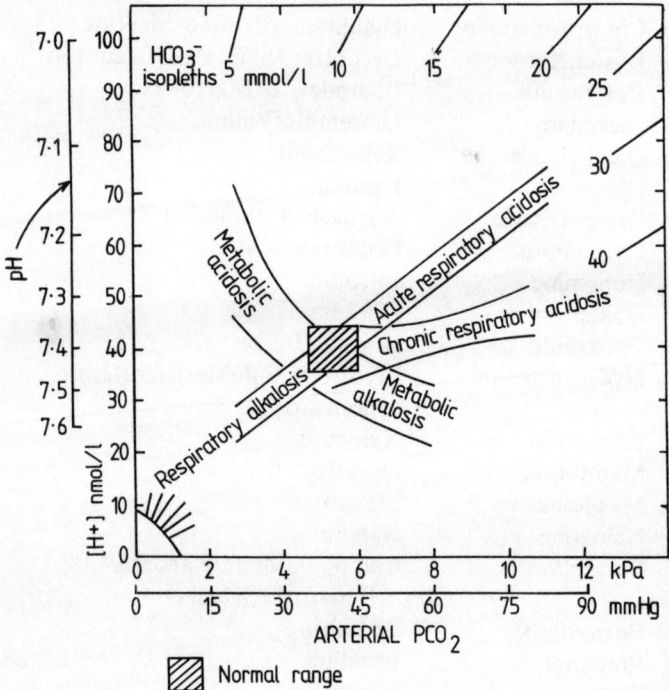

Fig. 24. Acid–base diagram (reproduced with permission from Flenley, D. C. (1971) *Lancet* i, 921)

POISONS INFORMATION CENTRES

National centre	Telephone number
Belfast	0232 40503
Cardiff	0222 569200
Dublin	0001 745588
Edinburgh	031 229 2477
London	01 407 7600

Non-national centre	Telephone number
Leeds	0532 430715
Manchester	061 795 7000
Newcastle	0632 325131

BIBLIOGRAPHY

TEXTBOOKS

Accident and Emergency Medicine. Edited by: Rutherford, W. H., Nelson, P. G., Weston, P. A. M., Wilson, D. H. Pitman Medical: London, 1980.

An Introduction to Electrocardiography. Schamroth, L. Blackwell Scientific: Oxford, 1978.

Casualty Radiology. Grech, P. Chapman & Hall: London, 1981.

Chest Injuries. Keen, G. John Wright: Bristol, 1977.

Diagnosis and Management of Acute Poisoning. Proudfoot, A. T. Blackwell Scientific: Oxford, 1982.

Emergency Medicine. Evans, R. Butterworths: London, 1981.

Management of Head Injuries. Jennett, B. and Teasdale, G. F. A. Davis: Philadelphia, 1981.

Practical Fracture Management. McRae, R. Churchill Livingston: Edinburgh, 1981.

Shock Trauma Manual. Gill, W. and Long, B. Williams and Wilkins: Baltimore, 1979.

Symposium on Burns. The Surgical Clinics of North America, Vol. 58, No. 6. W. B. Saunders: London, Philadelphia, 1978.

Trauma. Edited by: Carter, D. C. and Polk, H. C. Butterworths: London, 1981.

ARTICLES

Acute severe asthma. Editorial. *Lancet*, 1981, **i**, 313.

Aspects of the management of shock. Shine, K. I. *Ann. Intern. Med.* 1980, **93**, 723–734.

Diagnostic difficulties and problems in assessment of blunt chest injuries. Glinz, W. In: *Care of the Acutely Ill and Injured*. Edited by: Wilson, D. H. and Marsden, A. K. John Wiley & Sons: Chichester, 1982.

Early management of head injuries. Cockard, H. A. *Br. J. Hosp. Med.* 1982, **27/6**, 635–644.

Endotracheal intubation. Jones, D. F. *Hospital Update*, 1979, **5/12**, 1107–1117.

Hypothermia in the elderly. Emslie-Smith, D. *Br. J. Hosp. Med.* 1981, **26/5**, 442–452.

Problems of immersion. Golden, F. St.C. *Br. J. Hosp. Med.* 1980, **23/4**, 371–383.

Standards and guidelines for cardiopulmonary resuscitation and emergency cardiac care. *J.A.M.A.* 1980, **244**, **5**, 453–509.

The Heimlich maneuver. Heimlich, H. J. and Uhley, M. H. *Ciba Clinical Symposia*, 1979, **31**, 3.

The pathophysiology of shock. Ledingham, I. McA. and Routh, G. S. *Br. J. Hosp. Med.* 1979, **22/5**, 472–482.

INDEX

178